LIVES ON THE EDGE

TUBERCULOSIS in Marginalised Populations

Radheshyam Jadhav

SPEAKING
TIGER

SPEAKING TIGER BOOKS LLP
125A, Ground Floor, Shahpur Jat, near Asiad Village,
New Delhi 110049

First published by Speaking Tiger Books 2022

Copyright © Radheshyam Jadhav 2022

ISBN 978-93-5447-210-7
eISBN 978-93-5447-202-2

10 9 8 7 6 5 4 3 2 1

All rights reserved.
No part of this publication may be reproduced, transmitted,
or stored in a retrieval system, in any form or by any means,
electronic, mechanical, photocopying, recording or otherwise,
without the prior permission of the publisher.

This book is sold subject to the condition that it shall not,
by way of trade or otherwise, be lent, resold, hired out,
or otherwise circulated, without the publisher's prior
consent, in any form of binding or cover other
than that in which it is published.

Radheshyam Jadhav is an award-winning journalist and communication researcher with over 20 years of experience in field reporting. He holds a PhD in journalism and communication science and has been a British Chevening Gurukul fellow at the LSE. A two-time winner of the prestigious Ramnath Goenka Excellence in Journalism Award, he has also been an Asia Journalism Fellow at the Nanyang Technological University, Singapore.

Radheshyam has won several prestigious awards and fellowships, including the Statesman Award for Rural Reporting. With a proven track record of writing about politics, gender issues, health, agriculture, environment, and rural and urban development issues, his research in journalism and communication has been based on field visits. He has covered socio-economic and political stories extensively while working with national newspapers such as *The Hindu BusinessLine*, *The Times of India*, and *The Indian Express*. He has also contributed to academia in various capacities and is an adjunct professor at Vishwakarma University, Pune. His recently published books are *Harvesting Hope in the Suicide Zone* and *Trail of the Tiger—Uddhav Balasaheb Thackeray*.

To
The Brave Ones of the Survivors Against TB
(SATB) Movement
&
My dear friend, late Mohan Maskar-Patil

CONTENTS

Acknowledgements ix
Foreword xiii
Introduction xix
Author's Note xxv

1. Infants and TB: No Fairy Tale — 2
2. Teenagers and TB: A Long Run — 15
3. Deprivation and TB: Sunanda's Spine — 29
4. Livelihood and TB: Rolling Death — 44
5. Abandoned Women and TB: A Lonely Battle — 58
6. Faith and TB: God's Curse — 70
7. Transgenders and TB: Trapped Souls — 83
8. Nutrition and TB: Living on Rats — 97
9. Tribals and TB: The Trail — 112

10. Migration and TB: The Unending Quest   128

11. Stigma and TB: Myths and Reality   142

12. Covid-19 Pandemic and TB: 156
    A Dual Burden

Annexure   166

Acknowledgements

In March 2020, Survivors Against TB (SATB) awarded me a fellowship to write stories on poverty, undernutrition, and TB. Unfortunately, the Covid-19 outbreak and consequent lockdowns started soon after. Many members of my family were infected with Covid-19. I, too, suffered from the disease and had to be hospitalised. However, thanks to Dr Manish Kolge and Dr Dnyanesh Umalkar at Rao Nursing Home, Pune, I recovered and was able to commence work.

However, there were travel restrictions in place and I was unable to start any fieldwork. Indeed, there were times when I was not sure if I would be able to complete this project. But Chapal Mehra of SATB stood behind me like a rock during those testing times and allowed me to work at my convenience. The initial idea was to write a few stories for my newspaper, but during my discussions with Chapal, we felt a book would work better and he asked me to go ahead. My deepest thanks to Chapal and my friends at SATB.

As I started working, discussions with my co-fellow Shruti Jain helped a lot. SATB members extended all their support. During my travels in the field, many good Samaritans facilitated my journey. I am grateful to Aniket Lohiya and Irfan Shaikh of Manavlok (Beed), Suresh Nakhate (Nashik), Anuradha Kadam, Sadhana Zadbuke, Deepa Shipurkar, Anuradha Bhosale (Kolhapur), Suryakant Asbe (Solapur), and Sanyogita Dhamdhere (Pune).

Raghuvir Srinivasan, my editor at *The Hindu BusinessLine* provided me with a great deal of support and encouragement. Thomas K. Thomas and Lokeshwarri S.K., too, have been a constant support. I also thank my former editors at *The Times of India*—Jaideep Bose, Rohit Saran, Shankar Raghuraman, Vikas Singh, and Joy Purkayastha as well as my friend Atul Thakur for their constant support. Professor Dr. Siddharth Jabade, Vice-Chancellor, Vishwakarma University Pune, Professor Dr. Wasudeo Gade, Vice-President, Vishwakarma University, and Professor Dr. Chetan Kapadnis have supported my research endeavours in all possible ways.

Without the support of my wife Ambika and son Siddharth, undertaking the journey of writing this book during the pandemic would have been impossible.

A. Shenoy, a former colleague and close friend, who has always encouraged my fieldwork, guided me during these testing times and also helped me to edit these stories.

Special thanks to Ravi Singh, publisher and co-founder of Speaking Tiger Books for publishing this book. I am also grateful to Vineetha Mokkil for editing the book and giving valuable suggestions.

Foreword

Until Covid-19 devastated India, TB was and remained its severest health crisis. As Covid-19 recedes and then reappears in its spread, TB remains devastating, killing over 1,200 Indians every day. As I read the stories in this book, I was reminded of my time as a TB patient. The everyday struggle, medicines with severe side effects, mood swings, and the fear of infecting others. This, when I was privileged and could get the best care available. My journey was easier but still not easy.

People often forget that TB can happen to anyone, not just those who are underprivileged and marginalised. We tend to believe in such stereotypes about TB and this feeds the existing misinformation and stigma. This is why *Lives on the Edge: Tuberculosis in Marginalised Populations* is critically important as it is a reminder that while

Covid-19 has disrupted life globally, TB continues to kill people in large numbers, especially those who are vulnerable. We are all at risk, each one of us.

TB was and continues to remain a problem of staggering proportions. This book with its in-depth research and moving human stories is an alarm bell sounding out how poverty, hunger, gender inequality, failing health systems, and now, Covid-19, make TB a deadlier crisis of even bigger proportions. The stories in this book are of those whom we all claim to work for—India's most vulnerable. Yet, these stories ask us a difficult question—have we done enough? The answer is a clear NO.

This book examines the lived experiences and narratives of TB-affected individuals, and documents the everyday and systemic challenges that they face. It also explores alternatives and ways ahead to address these epidemics collectively as India and the world come to terms with living with Covid-19. Every story and every voice counts.

Even today, our approach to TB remains mired in just diagnosis and treatment. We continue to neglect the lived experience and the socioeconomic determinants of TB. Why this apathy towards the more fundamental holistic approaches to population health?

There are other issues as well. TB remains highly stigmatised. The cultural ideas about TB associate it with socially unacceptable lifestyles and behaviours with particular reference to sexual behaviour, promiscuity, alcohol, smoking, and other 'sins'. Similarly, TB and mental health are deeply related, though often ignored. The global community and in particular, high-burden countries like India, are not talking or strategizing enough about them.

Gender disparities in TB are striking. While TB affects more men than women, the brunt of social stigma disproportionately impacts women. Moreover, trans individuals, non-binaries, and persons with non-heteronormative sexual orientations are less likely to report their condition as they face discrimination and abuse by healthcare authorities, and are often given poor quality care or denied access to it altogether on account of their gender and/or sexual identities. These conditions are exacerbated for those seeking care for TB and living with HIV.

As health systems both globally and in India have put in efforts into managing the Covid-19 pandemic, they have diverted focus, personnel, critical resources, and health services for diseases other than Covid-19. A key impacted disease is TB where detection, treatment, awareness, and access to TB care have all fallen. The media headlines have all been about Covid-19 and the impending crisis and how it has devastated our population, economy, freedom, and minds. Forgotten in this uproar are numerous other diseases like TB that continue to devastate India's population.

Despite an extensive national programme and a vast private sector, India continues to bear the highest burden of TB in the world, accounting for an estimated 2.8 million cases every year and killing more than 4,00,000 people. Additionally, a growing burden of drug-resistant TB (DR-TB) threatens all the progress made in basic TB control. India's TB problem is increasingly considered a global problem.

Behind these figures are stories of lakhs of TB patients who die each year. TB is so widespread that it not just destroys lives, but also pushes millions into poverty and debt. This happens even when its more dangerous forms such as DR-TB remain curable.

What do the stories in this book tell us? Despite all our calls to action, even today, TB services remain widely uneven leading to delays in diagnosis, treatment, access, and possibly increased suffering and mental health issues for those affected. What then is the impact, implications, and possibilities that exist for addressing this ancient epidemic?

The Covid-19 pandemic and the impact it has on TB presents an opportunity to improve access to health services, innovative tools, and strategies, and community-based interventions that have been ignored for too long. Access is critical for eliminating TB and other diseases as it ensures early diagnosis and treatment and also equitable care. Some cannot afford tests and treatment while others are caught somewhere between an overburdened government system and a profit-driven private sector to access tests and treatment. Existing delivery approaches in the health system will need to be adapted as the risk-benefit analysis for any given activity changes in the context of a pandemic.

The challenges around treatment for TB are severe. We need to ensure that every patient is traced and tested and provided free, high-quality treatment, made available at their doorstep. We also have to provide patients education in their local language.

The time for slogans is over. The need is for political and financial commitment to ensure availability and easy accessibility of these tests and drugs to all TB patients. The State also needs to work with the private sector, which is accountable for providing access and ensuring essential tests and drugs are in supply and available at affordable prices. To do this, the government must work to create a relationship of mutual trust.

This book is a wakeup call to the entire health system, which disregards the needs of those struggling with diseases like TB. When it comes to infectious diseases like Covid-19 and TB, if we ignore even one patient, not only do we risk lives, we risk the spread of TB and Covid-19 as well. This is both unacceptable and inhuman. Even one life lost to TB is one too many.

PRIYA DUTT
Politician, former Member of Parliament, social worker, and TB survivor and advocate

Introduction

Almost eight years ago, I sat with Owais, one of India's earliest totally drug-resistant TB patients in the famous informal settlement of Dharavi. As he told me his story, in his one-room Dharavi home where he lived with his wife and two kids, the famous Mumbai rains arrived. At first, they were gentle, and then a torrent soaking the houses and filling the streets with their fury.

Owais, a slight man, weakened by HIV and drug-resistant TB, spoke to me haltingly about his battle against TB and his romance with Mumbai. He would pause and lean over, unable to speak louder. The rain outside beating on the neighbouring tin roofs and empty buckets did not help.

Owais was one of seven children in an agricultural family from Bihar. He migrated to Mumbai and fell in love with the city. He was an excellent tailor until TB and HIV happened to him. He mixes up dates and years but he knew that ever since he had got drug-resistant TB, life changed completely. He leaned over and asked me the moot question that vulnerable TB-affected individuals often ask, 'Why doesn't anyone care?' I hear this unerringly and often.

As I read through the stories in this book, put together by Radheshyam Jadhav, I am reminded of this question yet again. Over several years that we have worked on infectious diseases like TB, the attention to them has increased but resources are waning. Yet, those affected by TB do not understand this strange dichotomy and lack of engagement. Their lives remain devastated by this curable disease. They are often unable to go back to their old life or start a new one. They exist in limbo with their questions.

Covid-19 arrived and devastated our current system and exposed its lack of preparedness for dealing with infectious diseases. Yet, as Covid-19 recedes for now, we are back to asking the same things for TB as we did before Covid-19.

As we read the stories in this book, we are reminded again and again of the unaddressed challenges in TB that plague us even today. We are still asking for resources and change. These stories remind us of how little has changed and how far we have to go. India is still the global TB capital, home to over one-fourth of TB patients globally.

We have a growing population of drug-resistant TB cases that are hard to diagnose, and harder to treat. We are also credited with designing, implementing, and launching one of the world's largest TB control programmes. Why then, do we fail in addressing TB? Do we lack ability, innovative thinking, or just political attention and will?

India has close to 2.8 million new TB cases each year. This has probably risen during the pandemic. Behind these statistics are real people, their lives, and families that are devastated by this disease, struggling and fighting—asking the same question.

Many, including India's former Health Minister, termed TB a national emergency. They were all absolutely right but this rarely translated into action. More recently, Covid-19 changed our world. We all struggled, grieved, and suffered. TB was amongst the worst affected in services and attention. And we were back struggling with TB where we were decades ago.

So, what transformation can we ask for to make the lives of those affected by TB better? The stories in this book provide us some important lessons if we listen. Let us start with the basics. We still lack the ability to provide basic quality diagnosis and treatment unfailingly to TB patients. They struggle from pillar to post to get an accurate diagnosis. We lack machines and cartridges. We lack access. Whether in the public or private sector. Even today, our efforts to update diagnostics in the public sector and ensure access in the private sector remain well behind our needs. India needs to urgently invest extensively in diagnostics, including mobile testing, but most people have to travel miles to get a test.

Treatment is no different. People are still struggling to get the right treatment. The public sector has stockouts and the private sector often could not care less. The TB drug pipelines for both basic and advanced anti-TB drugs are often unreliable. The hardest hit are children with shortages of pediatric drugs or those within the public sector, where accountability is low.

As the stories in this book illustrate, an underlying and ignored aspect is that of poverty and resulting undernutrition. If we continue to test and treat for TB without food security, nutritional support, and guidance, we are chasing a mirage. TB will never be controlled, leave alone eliminated. There are other issues of urbanization, where our poor migrate to cities and then live in overcrowded, unsanitary conditions where there is no proper waste management. This, combined with heavy air pollution and undernutrition, is a tinderbox for feeding the flames of TB.

Even nutritional support programmes remain plagued with problems. The Nikhay Poshan Yojana amount remains insufficient and mired in paperwork often never reaching TB-affected individuals even after treatment. Why should that be the case? Because the system is designed to delay and dismiss the needs of those that remain vulnerable. A critical question, as the stories in this book show, is the experience of care as per gender. We need gender-sensitive care as defined by diverse gender and sexual identities. Yet, this participative model remains a far cry and these groups remain on the fringes stigmatised by the health system itself.

TB may have been an ancient killer but because its primary problems are linked to age-old determinants—poverty, class, gender, caste, and human rights—we stereotype, stigmatise, and dismiss those affected from our collective conscience. We justify it by saying they must be doing something to deserve it—or rather, 'they brought it upon themselves'. Even today, the TB-affected remain highly stigmatised, sometimes losing their social status, employment, and even their dignity in the fight against TB. They suffer quietly; denied care, taunted, and made to feel grateful for poor quality care which ideally, should be unacceptable.

Despite all this, TB still lacks the political attention and consequently the funding or the innovative thinking that it needs. Instead, we get empty slogans that further dilute the ethical responsibility of the State. It is a cruel irony that Covid-19 that devastated the world and saw endless funding remains incurable whereas TB has been curable for decades, and yet, is fighting for the attention it needs. In India, the affected people—the vulnerable minorities, are still asking for the basics of what they deserve from the State: correct diagnosis and treatment, nutritional support, dignity and support without paternalism, and stigma-free care.

I still remember when we ended our interview with Owais. Sitting on the floor of his home, Owais smiled and told me that he was grateful he was alive to see his children. As the rain began to fall relentlessly over Dharavi, the family sat together on the floor. His daughter pored over a book. Owais and his son went and sat by the doorway, to watch the rain envelop Mumbai. The question in the air remained, 'Do lives affected by TB matter?'

CHAPAL MEHRA
Public health specialist, writer, and convenor,
Survivors Against TB

Author's Note

'First, treat us as human beings and then treat our disease,' were Soumya's last words when our conversation ended. She was being treated for HIV and tuberculosis (TB), and her health was deteriorating. It has been thirteen years and I do not know what happened to her or where she is. I met her for the first and last time in 2008, in Koovagam village, Tamil Nadu, during an annual festival. She refused to remain in contact. Soumya had lost faith in the outer world and wanted to live quietly in her community. She was not bothered by the discrimination and stigma she faced from having HIV and TB. As a transgender, she had suffered much more. For her and many others in India's marginalised communities, TB is not just a disease.

There is graded prejudice, discrimination, and isolation related to TB and its corrosive impact intensifies and multiplies when the patient hails from a marginalised community. Marginalisation is the deprivation of people, communities, and groups—the exercise of control over their resources and lives, preventing them from becoming part of the development story. Here, I define development as qualitative and quantitative advancement in socio-economic-political structures for the betterment of human life. Development with dignity is based on the premise of justice (social, economic, and political), liberty (of thought, expression, belief, faith, and worship), equality (of status and opportunity), and fraternity (the dignity of the individual).

People are marginalised mainly because of gender, caste, class, creed, race, and sexual orientation. Marginalisation is a process of disempowerment and people experience it in different ways. But even marginalisation is understood from an androcentric perspective, which is a male-centred view and explanation of the concept.

Among members of marginalised communities, TB comes with a huge burden. And if the patient is a woman or an LGBTQ community member, the suffering multiplies at every level. From stigma to discrimination and diagnosis to treatment, they experience marginalisation in different ways. They are part of the lowest strata of society and family. Women and LGBTQ members in marginalised communities are the worst affected. They are marginalised even among the marginalised.

The TB Tales

The majority of stories in this book build a narrative about the daunting challenges a woman has to face when she is diagnosed with TB. A ten-month-old baby girl is already an unwanted member of the house (because of her gender), and TB just adds to the reasons why she is shunned. A teenager who dreams of winning a medal for India in the Olympics fights back when infected with TB, but the main worry for her family and society is her marriage. Sunanda is a coordinator at the antiretroviral therapy (ART) department at the government hospital in Kolhapur and was married off by her father at fifteen. She contracted HIV from her husband and has had to thereafter fight TB all alone. Women in Solapur inhale tobacco, suffer TB, and cough blood but have to continue bidi rolling to earn a livelihood for their families. There are many who are abandoned by their husbands after being infected. 'God's women' or devadasis suffer brutal exploitation and live in denial of HIV and TB. Transgenders still remain social pariahs, with nobody bothering about their lives and health. Musahars, the Mahadalits whose socio-economic life is worse than that of Dalits, still struggle to eat two meals a day, while politicians debate whether starvation or TB is responsible for their deaths. Tribal communities, meanwhile, are far away from the TB healthcare system and the system is unaware of how women suffer and die from TB in remote areas.

Other stories deal with migrants—the 'TB carriers'—who suffered the most during the Covid-19 pandemic. TB infections amid the pandemic added to their mental distress, the impact of which will be long-lasting. The stigma associated with TB has destroyed many a family.

India's TB Burden

Tuberculosis remains one of the most critical health challenges in India, with severe socio-economic and cultural consequences for patients and their families. India has the largest burden of TB globally in terms of absolute numbers, with an estimated 2.64 million patients. The Government of India has developed a National Strategic Plan (2017-25) to eradicate TB in India by 2025. The key focus areas of this plan include early diagnosis of all TB patients, prompt treatment with quality-assured drugs, along with suitable patient-support systems to promote adherence. The government is also engaging with patients seeking care in the private sector. Prevention strategies include active case detection and contact tracing in high-risk/vulnerable populations. A multi-sectoral response to address social determinants is also part of the plan.

However, the ground reality is grim. Government plans and schemes are yet to reach the last woman standing in the line. Structures become more and more redundant and exploitative as they trickle down to the marginalised. A more humane approach is necessary when it comes to TB treatment of these sections. Not only the government and private health machinery, but society as a whole must change their attitudes and approaches towards TB patients from marginalised communities. But that seems a distant dream as TB remains taboo even among the educated and the elite classes.

Why These Stories?

The stories based on field visits draw attention to the grassroots reality. Three stories in this book: Koovagam—2008, Kushinagar—2018, and Solapur—2017, are based on field visits I had made earlier. The other nine stories are part of field visits I made while working on the Survivors Against TB (SATB) fellowship in 2020-21. I have also used information and data collected over the years during my reporting.

But these stories are not just heartbreaking tales

about how TB affects marginalised communities. During my field trips, I also came across individuals and community members fighting their battles with grit and determination, and going all out to improve their lives. So, there is a silver lining to their stories as well.

Shailaja Narwade is sowing seeds of change in an area where girls are unwanted. TB-infected teenager Aki is scripting an incredible story of resilience and sporting excellence. Sunanda has come out in the open to declare herself an HIV and TB patient, saying that it is not taboo to be a patient. Bidi rollers in Solapur are making efforts to build healthy accommodation for themselves. Women in drought-prone areas are becoming health conscious and saving up for their medical treatment.

Musahar Ramrati Devi put up a brave fight to save her land so that the next generation does not have to starve and is fit to fight any disease. Living in the remote Kombhalne village in Maharashtra's Ahmednagar district, Rahibai Popere is trying to address malnourishment. Young people who migrated to cities and returned to villages during the Covid-19 pandemic are experimenting with farming so that they do not have to go back and live in congested city slums, which are TB dens.

SATB members have been sharing their TB experience widely on various platforms. Their stories have helped many TB patients deal with the disease and issues such as stigma and discrimination. The Covid-19 pandemic has taught many lessons and communities have come forward to help the needy.

TB is much more than an infection and a disease and these stories reflect this ground reality. I am sure that this effort will help those who want to understand TB better from the grassroots perspective.

RADHESHYAM JADHAV

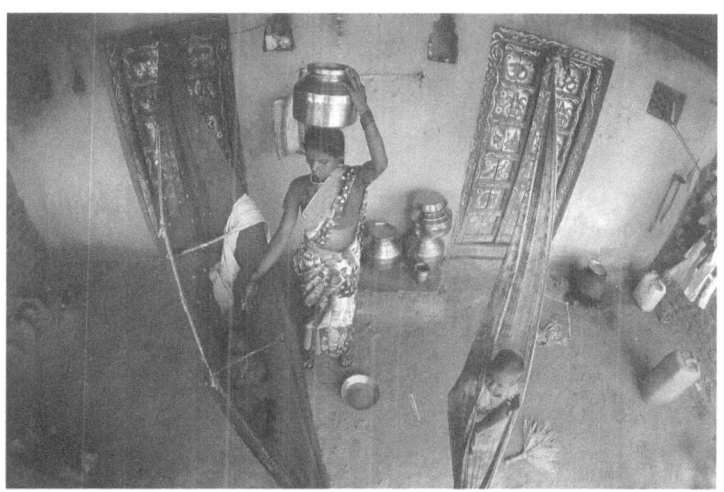

Poor parents fear that the tag 'TB baby' would haunt the child forever, especially girls, and marrying them off would be difficult. *(representative image. picture credit: Deshpande M)*

1

Infants and TB: No Fairy Tale

When Simran (name changed) realised she was pregnant, she was neither excited nor happy. The first thought that came to her mind was whether it would be a girl or a boy. This mattered most because her life and her child's entire future depended on this. She told her husband that she was pregnant. He was excited at the thought that now there would be a son to continue the family name and look after them in their dotage. He did not even consider the fact that the child could be a girl.

With the threat of the Covid-19 pandemic growing more severe, the health machinery in Beed district in the Marathwada region of Maharashtra was kept on its toes. The health sector in Maharashtra, which was the worst Covid-19 affected State in India, was receiving a lot of attention. Moreover, the frequent media focus on sex determination/selection and induced abortions in Beed had put some pressure on medical practitioners who indulged in such practices. While these practices still continue despite various laws as well as non-governmental organizations' (NGOs') efforts to end them, the practitioners have become cautious and now demand more money. People living in rural areas tend to believe that contraceptive pills are not very reliable.

Married at a young age, this was Simran's first pregnancy and she knew that more would follow. Women in the region are forced to have children till they bear a son or the desired number of sons. This preference for male children leads to them having many children. Both women and men want more sons than daughters. In 2019, Beed was in the news because a migrant labourer who had been pregnant twenty times had given birth to her seventeeth baby. The woman has eleven children, nine of whom are girls. She had gone for three abortions while five of her children had died.

Pune-based Gokhale Institute of Politics and Economics released a study on Shirur Kasar village of Beed district in 2013. The study revealed that societal acceptance of sex determination and selection and induced abortions is on the rise. As per the 2011 census, the district had a dismal sex ratio of 801 girls for every 1,000 boys. In 2001, it was 894 girls for every 1,000 boys. Shirur Kasar had the lowest child sex ratio in the State—it was 955 in 1991 and fell to 768 in 2011. The project report concluded that women have undergone repeated abortions despite being aware that they could face health problems. Experts say that one of the main reasons for the lopsided child sex ratio is discrimination against females, worsened by a low total fertility rate (the number of children a woman bears in her lifetime).[1]

About 82.3% of women and 83% of men across all categories want at least one son in the family, according to the National Family Health Survey 2015-16. Across States, 18.8% of women and 19.2% of men want more sons than daughters. Only 3.5% of the women and the men in India want more daughters than sons. Daughters are still considered 'a burden', and a 'glass vessel' that can crack easily and bring disrepute to the family. A daughter is a 'responsibility'; she is 'others' property' and someone who cannot become an old-age support for her parents. Whatever she earns will go into her husband's or in-laws' pockets and not to her parents.[2]

Not surprisingly, Simran was under pressure to deliver a baby boy. 'Society believes that boys are better than girls. We don't really think this. But how could society be wrong?' asks Simran's father, a daily-wage worker. He married off Simran to a boy who is a daily-wage earner like him.

'Once a girl is married, her life is set,' said the father. He meant that once she starts having children, she will get busy with her life. Simran had no choice in the matter. She married according to her father's wishes and lived her life as per her husband's will. But even after marriage, her father had to shoulder her delivery expenses, according to the tradition of the region. Simran was desperately praying for a boy, but her worst fears came true and she delivered a baby girl.

TB Baby

The family was dismayed and the baby was now Simran's and her father's responsibility. As she started feeding the baby, Simran realised that the baby was not digesting food properly and was throwing up at times. Even after nine months, the baby's weight had not increased and the mother feared that the baby had Covid-19. Simran's father decided to take the child for a check-up.

Initially, her family members were unwilling to go for a check-up, but the baby's condition was deteriorating. Simran's father took her to the Primary Health Centre (PHC) in the town and the doctors there recommended some tests. The baby was diagnosed with a latent TB infection. TB bacteria were found in the body but the baby was not sick and had no symptoms of the disease. Many people with a latent TB infection do not necessarily develop the disease but in some cases the bacteria can multiply and result in the disease.

Latent Tuberculosis Infection (LTBI) is defined as a state of persistent immune response to stimulation by Mycobacterium tuberculosis antigens with no evidence of clinically manifest active TB, states a WHO document. There is no gold standard for direct identification of Mycobacterium tuberculosis infection in humans. Most infected people have no signs or symptoms of TB but are at risk of active tuberculosis. The document highlights that infants aged less than twelve months, living with HIV, and in contact with a TB carrier, should receive six months of Isoniazid Preventive Treatment (IPT) if an investigation shows no TB. All infants less than one year of age should be given preventive treatment if they have a history of household contact with a TB case, adds the document, titled 'Latent Tuberculosis Infection'.[3]

'No. Not at all. We don't have any family history of TB or other diseases. I don't know how the baby got TB. It is surprising and a shock for all of us,' says Simran's father. After further discussion, he reveals that his brother had contracted TB a few years earlier. 'But that has nothing to do with the baby's TB,' he insists.

The PHC medical supervisor observing the baby's treatment says that the family found it hard to digest the fact that the baby had TB. 'They feared that people and their relatives would call the child a TB baby and the tag would haunt her forever. The family has not informed relatives and neighbours about the baby's TB infection. Instead, they say she has a stomach problem and is being treated for it,' says the supervisor.

Simran's husband and his family are agitated. Their expectations of having a baby boy had not been fulfilled and the birth of a girl with TB had filled them with disgust. Even if a child is born handicapped, it is considered okay as this is accepted by society. But TB is a stigma, says the family, which is making every possible effort to conceal the information. The family members do not want PHC officials and workers coming to their house for visits. They have also requested hospital employees not to reveal the diagnosis to anyone. In their small town, the TB infection would result in a social boycott, they fear. TB and leprosy are the same for many people in the town, as awareness and understanding about TB is very low.

The medical supervisor has told the family that TB is curable and that the baby will recover completely in six months. 'But don't miss the medicine timetable. Regular medicine should go into the baby's stomach,' he has warned the family members. The family has informed him that every possible care is being taken. They had only missed the medicine a couple of times.

Simran dilutes tablets in water and honey and gives them to the baby. She and her family fear that the child will have a TB relapse later in life and that this would create problems when she got married.

'The only important event in the life of a girl here is marriage and not her education, career, and development. The moment a girl is born, her parents start saving for her marriage and dowry. This mentality has ruined the lives of thousands of girls in the region,' says Beed-based activist Manisha Tokale.

Sheetal, a teenager from Pimpla village in the district, was married to a farmer called Dadasaheb Toge. But she kept returning to her parents' house. She wanted to go to school and play with her friends. Sheetal was just one among many minors being forced to tie the knot in the region. 'She wouldn't listen,' her father told the police. One day, Sheetal's body was found in the fields. The police allege that her father strangled her. Activists believe that farm distress, escalated by the financial difficulties posed by Covid-19, has led to an increase in the number of marriages of minors. 'Visit Marathwada's villages, and you will find at least 4-5 cases of child marriages during the pandemic,' says Tatvasheel Kamble, a member of Beed's Child Welfare Committee.

For many like Sheetal and Simran, being a girl is a curse. Sheetal is no more, and Simran's baby is a 'TB Girl'. Simran cries day and night thinking about what will happen to her little girl.

Nakushi—The Unwanted

In many parts of Maharashtra, newborn baby girls are named Nakushi and Dhonda. 'Nakushi' means unwanted and 'Dhonda' means stone or a burden. Many girls in drought-affected areas have these names, with their families grudgingly accepting their existence. Right from birth, they are told that they are unwanted and this tag stays with them forever. These girls rarely get to go to school. When they do, it is not for long. Kalpana Chambulwar from Wardha district of Vidarbha says that when the drought becomes severe, almost all girls abandon school in search of water. 'Here, girls are born to fetch water and do farm work. From childhood till death, we have to do the same work,' she explains. Apart from fetching water, women work as unpaid labourers in their own farms as the farmland is owned by men.

One of the questions the medical supervisor monitoring Simran's baby's treatment faces from villagers is whether TB in women affects their ability to work. 'Life is not easy for girls here,' he says, drawing attention to news about the deaths of girls and women while fetching water from wells during the summer. 'Come drought and you will find such news,' he adds. There are thousands of girls traversing parched landscapes searching for water in the region, where drought is perennial. The responsibility of fetching water for the household rests solely on women and girls.

Simran's family, too, fears that TB will affect the child's marriage and physical capacity to work. 'What will the future of my child be?' is the only question Simran asks. Nobody has an answer.

Heralding Change

'There are no easy answers to such questions in this region. It's a fight to survive from day one,' says Shailaja Narwade, a farmer and an entrepreneur from the neighbouring Masla village in Osmanabad district, who took the lead to establish the Vijayalaxmi Sakhi Producer Company. The company produces and markets pulses. She as well as other women also operate a seed business they launched during the Covid-19 pandemic.

Shailaja says that women in the region have to find their own answers. 'Change will not happen suddenly. We didn't get a chance to educate ourselves. But we will educate our girls. Now, it is high time that women claim ownership of land and take control of agriculture. Our land is our resource and a key to change the lives of our girls. Even women who are landless are part of our Producer Company.' Shailaja adds that girls should be educated, receive proper nourishment, and lead healthy lives. This is possible only if women earn a livelihood and take control of resources, she insists. Shailaja and others like her are inspiring Simran and many other women. Shailaja and her friends look at agriculture as a profit-making venture, using local resources and innovative ideas.

While tabling the 2017-18 Economic Survey in parliament, late Union Finance Minister Arun Jaitley had said that with the rise in rural to urban migration by men, 'feminisation' of the agriculture sector was taking root. He talked about how an increasing number of women were moving into multiple roles as cultivators, entrepreneurs, and labourers.

During the Covid-19 pandemic, more women in Marathwada moved into cultivation, pre-harvest work, post-harvest processing, packaging, and marketing activities. Amidst the crisis caused by Covid-19, these parts of rural Maharashtra are becoming a laboratory for the feminisation of agriculture. During the pandemic, men who had migrated to cities lost their jobs and returned to their villages. While men are going back to agriculture because of Covid-19, women are finding new ways to make agriculture a business through producer companies. There are many Shailajas today who are fighting battles for themselves and their daughters.

For Simran and her infant, the battle has just begun. The child is now ten months old and responding to treatment. However, there are questions over the family's commitment towards continuing the treatment and helping the baby recover completely. Simran and her baby are not just fighting TB—they are fighting family, society, tradition, stigma, and poverty. And the will to fight is the only weapon Simran has on hand in this arduous battle.

NOTES

1. Jadhav, R. (2013). 'More efforts needed to curb sex determination'. Retrieved from https://timesofindia.indiatimes.com/city/pune/more-efforts-needed-to-curb-sex-determination/articleshow/26014729.cms
2. Ministry of Health and Family Welfare. (2015-16). National Family Health Survey 2015-16. Retrieved from http://rchiips.org/nfhs/nfhs-4Reports/India.pdf
3. World Health Organization. (2018). Latent tuberculosis infection. Retrieved from https://apps.who.int/iris/bitstream/handle/10665/260233/9789241550239-eng.pdf

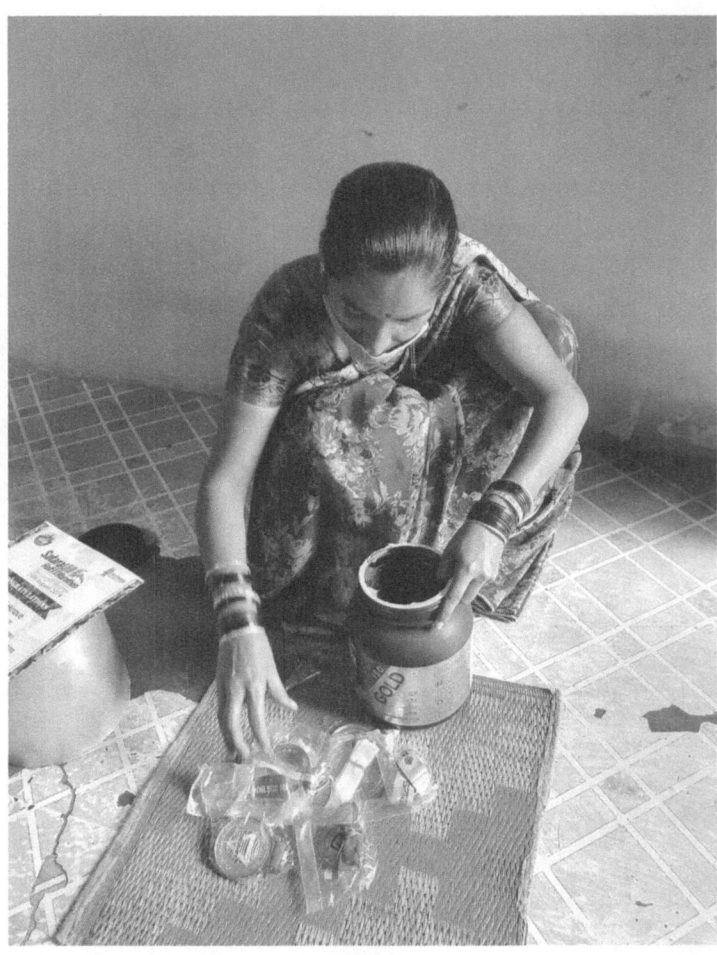

Aki's mother displays her daughter's medals. She wants to see Aki wearing India's blazer with a tricolour at the Olympics.
(picture credit: Radheshyam Jadhav)

2

Teenagers and TB: A Long Run

Aki (name changed) was thrilled to be back on the running track. It had been almost 3-4 months since she had come to the track and she had been desperately waiting for this moment. Despite her parents and sports teacher asking her not to do so, Aki was gearing up to run a taluka-level marathon. At age fourteen, she had already earned a reputation in Satara district (Maharashtra) and within the sports fraternity of the State. But this time, she had to prove herself again. Not to the world, but to herself. She was confident of winning the race. After all, it was just a thirty-four-metre track and she had completed more difficult marathons than this one. But at that moment, she kept all her laurels aside and focused on running the race. Her dream was at stake.

The fact that she hailed from a poor family in a remote, hilly village in Satara district did not deter Aki from dreaming big. A local school teacher had given wings to her dreams. The young teacher himself had wanted to be an athlete but could not fulfil his dream because of the lack of training and infrastructure. But when he became a teacher in the village, he decided to train his students in athletics. The terrain was hilly and there was no playground. Developing a running track was impossible because of the topography. The teacher requested the villagers to help him by allowing him to develop a running track on a small plateau. Some villagers cultivated the area during the monsoon and the land was barren otherwise. After much discussion, the villagers allowed him to develop the track. However, he had no money and resources, and hence the running track was nothing but plain, muddy ground. He started talking to the parents about athletics and told them to support their children as it held the promise of a future for them. The parents were not enthusiastic, but the students responded.

The teacher knocked on the doors of some small business houses, donors, and philanthropists in Satara and other parts of the State to help the students source shoes and dress material. However, the villagers insisted that girls would not be allowed to wear leggings, shorts, and T-shirts and could only run in traditional Punjabi clothing. And so it began. Soon, many people from villages came to see what athletics was all about. As the days passed, the girls resolved that they would wear leggings, shorts, and T-shirts as it was not possible to run in the cumbersome Punjabi attire. Parents opposed this, and the villagers said it would set a wrong precedent. A few parents, however, did allow their girls to go ahead and then people thronged the ground to see girls in shorts and T-shirts with their own eyes!

The teacher and his students came in for criticism from all corners. The students were told to concentrate on their studies and not get into such a 'circus'. But some parents and their kids were convinced and had confidence in the teacher. Aki's parents were among them.

Aki's father has a small cutlery shop near the village temple and also works as a contractor, putting up pandals (tents) during marriages and other ceremonies in the village. His wife chips in and also works as a cook at village functions like marriages. Aki's father does not make much money except during the annual fair of the village Goddess, when thousands of pilgrims flood the village. With three daughters and a son, he is not able to provide very well for his family. When Aki told her father that she wanted to join the group of girls who were being trained by the sports teacher, he did not oppose or support her.

But Aki won strong support from her mother, who was happy that her daughter was at least dreaming. Aki's mother was in the ninth standard when she was married off and her husband had hardly been to school. The mother had wanted to complete her education and be on her own, but her parents had disallowed this. Now, she had decided to educate all her girls and fulfil their dreams.

As Aki started her training, her mother supported her in every possible way. She was happy that someone in the family was daring to dream. Otherwise, life had been a long series of compromises. As Aki started participating in local running competitions, her teacher asked the mother to improve her diet. The mother had saved some money and started providing Aki a healthy diet. Aki won a gold medal at the State-level marathon when she was in the seventh standard and then repeated the performance at the west zone national in Rajasthan, at the under-sixteen level. She won marathon after marathon and became a phenomenon. Her story fascinated everyone and her parents were proud. By this time, they had used up all their savings on her training, travel, diet, and other expenses. They were now ready to sell everything, including their tiny home, so that she could continue to run and achieve her dream of becoming a national-level athlete and run in the Olympics.

Aki was determined and focused on her destination. She was on the right track. But then came a major hurdle that posed a giant question mark over her dreams.

A Dream Halted

In 2016, Aki went to Assam for a training camp and had a severe fever. When she returned, she felt fatigued. She was treated by a local doctor for a fever, but did not recover even after a month. Meanwhile, she also lost weight. The worried parents took her to a city hospital. She was asked to go in for various medical tests. A chest X-ray revealed two dark spots in her lungs and Aki was diagnosed with TB. The doctors asked her to stop running immediately.

'She was strong, even when the doctors told her that she had TB. But she broke down when she was told to stop running. Aki said she would not stop practising at any cost. She was not ready even to listen to her teacher,' says her mother. But her body and lungs were not in consonance with her grit. Aki soon realised that she could not even walk at a fast pace.

After trying out treatments in local hospitals, her teacher contacted a business group that had sponsored Aki and other girls. The group connected them to a doctor in Mumbai. Aki's treatment started, but all she could think about was how her career would be affected. Would she be able to run again? Everyone was giving her confidence and affirmative answers. But she was not convinced. She wanted to go back to the track and test her own capacity. The doctors told her that she needed to be on medication for nine months. And during the first few months, they warned her against taking up any kind of exertion or running practice.

Aki's parents and teacher faced a dual challenge. They were worried about the reaction of the villagers to the TB, which could lead to discrimination against the child and the family. Secondly, they were worried about Aki's mental and physical health. They feared that she would spiral into depression once she stopped practising.

The Call of the Track

About four months after her treatment had commenced, Aki was back on the track. Her treatment was still on but she insisted that she wanted to run. She wanted to prove that she was fine and could continue her practice. The best way was to prove her confidence in a competition. Hearing the words, 'On your mark, get set, go!' thrilled her and she pushed herself to run. It was like a dream for Aki. She put in everything into the race, but within a few minutes, the other athletes left her behind and she was not able to keep up. She started gasping for breath and in the last phase, she felt that she would not even be able to complete the race. But she continued to run and managed to complete the race. Teary-eyed, she was not able to take it in. Her future seemed to have gone up in smoke. Aki, her parents, and her teacher had not realised the seriousness of her disease.

Her defeat on the track was difficult to digest. It stung to be a national winner and not be able to compete even in a local race. But Aki was not ready to compromise on her dreams. Despite her parents' and her teacher's opposition, she went on to participate in district-level competitions. The results were the same—Aki was struggling just to finish the races. She felt that it was the end of her career.

'It took some time for her to accept the facts. One day, I went to her home. Not only Aki but her parents were also devastated. By this time, news of her TB was spreading slowly and that had added to their worries. I realised that if she was away from the ground, she was going to suffer more. That day, I told her that we were going to resume her training,' says her teacher.

Aki had become weak as her treatment continued. Her teacher started with basic training and did not allow her to put pressure on her lungs. After over nine months, they went to the doctor for a check-up. There was good news. She was on the path to recovery and the doctor told her that she might be able to start running soon.

In 2017 Aki was back on the track. In 2018-19, she ran the Goa cross-country race and since then she has run in almost eight national competitions, winning four medals. While recounting the story of her gritty daughter, her mother breaks down.

Aki's mother and her teacher narrate the story of how she is practising hard. But there are no trophies, medals, and certificates on display in her house. When she is asked about this, her mother smiles and goes inside, returning with a big, black plastic can. She opens the can and out come the medals. In a few seconds, there is a pile of them. She then opens a cupboard and takes out a tattered file containing her daughter's certificates.

'She says that there is no need to display her medals unless she wins one in the Asian competition,' says Aki's mother, adding, 'Why Asian competition? She could also win in the Olympics. We want to see her wearing India's blazer with a tricolour at the Olympics.' She pauses to dab away her tears with the loose end of her sari.

Dreams Come True

Aki's parents stand firmly behind her. A local newspaper featured her success story and mentioned the fact that she had TB.

I ask her mother if I, too, could use her name

and picture in this piece. But her mother does not answer my question. When Aki's teacher says her name could be used, the mother hesitantly nods. But she is not convinced. She says that one of her daughters is married, while Aki and the other daughter have a long way to go. To help the family, Aki's younger sister, along with her mother, works as a cook. 'Educating and marrying girls are tough tasks,' she says.

'I hope TB does not become a problem in her career and marriage. After all, she is a girl,' the mother tells herself and looks up to seek acknowledgment. The teacher says, 'Don't worry. She is a brave girl. She has overcome many hurdles. Her future is bright.'

But deep down, even he is worried if the TB will recur or impact her running career. 'This year she will be 21 and she has a career till 27-28. Now, the focus is on training her for the international level. She has that capacity. But the main thing is to give her a good diet and the best possible training at the national level. I'm trying my best,' he says.

Aki is not at home. She is attending a training camp and her teacher will visit her soon. Aki's mother has prepared peanut laddus (sweets) for her. 'She needs a healthy diet. Not these peanuts,' says the teacher. 'Wait, wait. This is not all. I am bringing more,' the mother says and brings out a box full of almonds and cashew nuts. 'This time, I could only manage this much. Next time, I will send her more healthy stuff.'

There is hope and dismay in her eyes. 'My girl is really bright. She can win an Olympic medal for India. We are trying our best to do whatever is possible,' she says.

While training, Aki has continued her studies. She is in the second year of her Bachelor of Arts course. The teacher says that once she completes her graduation, he will contact government and sports officials so that she gets a government job from the sports quota to attain financial stability.

In the training camp in Nanded, Aki is completely focused on her training. Sometimes, TB still haunts her, but she has decided to ignore the past. Right now, she is not thinking of anything but the next competition. When you dream, you have to work hard to realise the dream, she believes.

'Initially, when I was told I had the disease, I was not able to understand what TB is all about. My mother was afraid. I realised the seriousness when it started affecting my work,' says Aki. 'It took some time. But I decided to be strong. I kept talking to my teacher and my mother. It helped a lot. They supported me all the way. Now, I don't have any fear and I am focusing on my career.'

Ask her about marriage and she becomes uneasy. After a while, she says, 'I don't have any time right now to think about marriage and all. I want to run in the Olympics.'

The WHO's roadmap towards ending TB in children and adolescents (second edition), released in 2018, states that adolescent TB patients often present with bacteriologically infectious disease typical among adults (e.g. with cavities seen on chest X-rays). Hence, it poses a high risk for transmission in 'congregate' settings whether it is schools or houses. The report talks about the unique challenges teenagers like Aki face because of peer pressure and fear of stigma. There are other challenges like increasing prevalence of co-morbidities such as HIV, and risky behaviour such as alcohol, substance, and tobacco use. The report highlights that the age group of 10-19 needs adolescent-friendly services which include relevant psychological support and least disruption in educational life. 'Age-disaggregated data on adolescent TB are not routinely collected and reported (i.e., among those who are in the 10-14 and 15-19 years age groups),' the report adds.

The WHO notes that access to TB prevention and care is severely lacking when it comes to children and adolescents. More than one million children under the age of fifteen fall ill with TB every year, and over half of them are not diagnosed and/or not reported. Lack of a sensitive diagnostic test and limited diagnostic capacity results in the highest proportion of 'missing children'. Less than one-third of eligible child household contacts of patients with TB receive TB preventive treatment.[1]

It is raining heavily in Aki's village and the running track is slushy and muddied. The teacher has built a tin shed hostel so that students can stay there when they are training. There is no synthetic track, no basic infrastructure, not even clothing or shoes. 'I keep telling myself that I should not fear any challenge. Dedication and will are enough to face challenges,' says Aki.

In August 2021, the Government of India welcomed the country's Tokyo Olympics medal winners with a grand ceremony at Ashoka Hotel in New Delhi. The ministers and officials there celebrated the win saying it was an incredible story of resilience and sporting excellence.

Hundreds and thousands like Aki are scripting incredible stories of resilience and sporting excellence. But their struggle is theirs alone. To gain recognition, they have to win medals at the highest levels, as the world is interested only in their success and not in the struggle behind their success.

Aki knows this and continues to run. She has overcome TB, but there are more hurdles ahead of her in the race of life.

NOTES

1. World Health Organization. (2018). Roadmap towards ending TB in children and adolescents. Retrieved from https://www.who.int/activities/ending-tb-in-children-and-adolescents

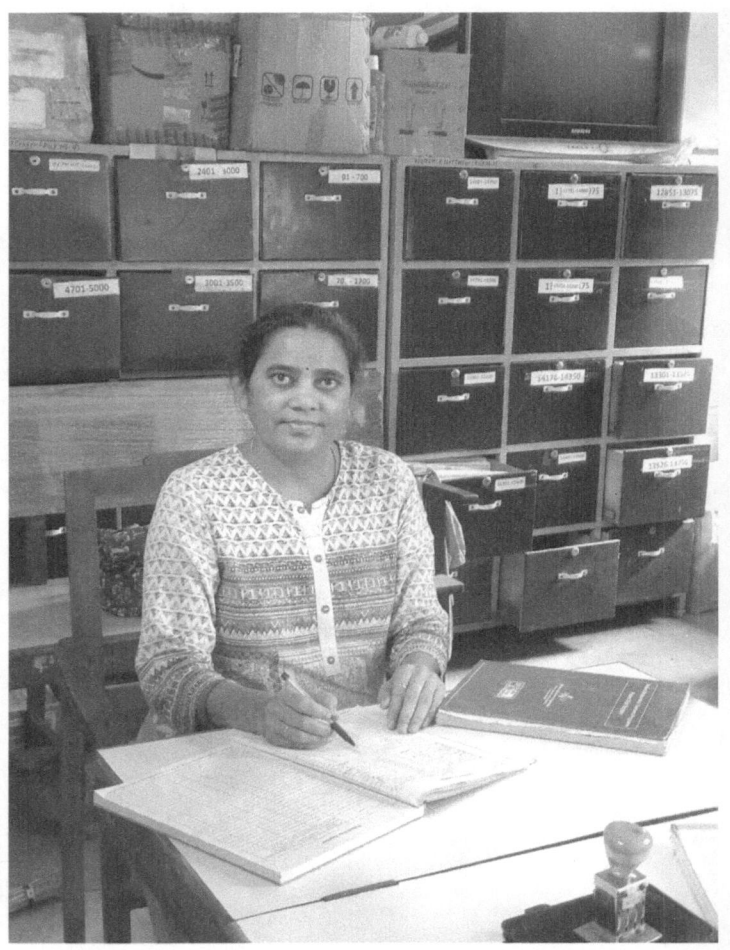

'What is there to hide in HIV and TB?' asks Sunanda, who battled both diseases and social stigma with sheer determination.
(picture credit: Radheshyam Jadhav)

3

Deprivation and TB: Sunanda's Spine

'Why suffer injustice? Why succumb to exploitation?' asks a visibly disturbed Sunanda. Sitting in a congested office room of a dark corridor in the Chhatrapati Pramila Raje Government Hospital in Kolhapur (Maharashtra), constructed way back in 1881, Sunanda goes silent for a few moments. She gazes through a window at the dark clouds hovering over the hospital, trying to hide her tears.

A couple enters the room and Sunanda immediately regains her composure. As the couple settles down in the chairs in her tiny office, Sunanda asks them, 'So, what have you decided?' The man and the woman look at each other and remain silent. Sunanda continues, 'Everyone has problems. But that doesn't stop us from living. Why should you not live a happy life? What is the problem? I am not just saying this to please you. I know it. Please go ahead and get married. Be happy. Don't be bothered by society and the world. We have discussed this even earlier and now you must take a call.'

The woman seems to be convinced but the man squirms in his chair. 'But there will be many problems. It will be difficult. I am not able to understand what I should do. Many times, I wonder why I should live at all. So, why get into marriage and all…what's the use?' he says. 'Not all marriages are successful. And in our case, it is unlikely to last long. Don't know when one of us will die,' he adds.

Sunanda smiles and offers him a glass of water. As he gulps the water, Sunanda says, 'Destiny has given you another chance to live. In fact, we have to fight to earn the right to live. Society is cruel. It will allow us to breathe but will ensure we cannot breathe. We have to fight.'

She has a story to tell and the couple is all ears. This is not the first couple to hear her story. For several years now, Sunanda has been sharing her tale with hundreds of people like them.

Gasping for Life

Sunanda's parents, hailing from Kasba Sangaon village in Kolhapur, planned to get her married when she was only fifteen. Her father, who was a sugarcane cutter, was finding it difficult to manage the family and wanted to get Sunanda out of his home as quickly as possible. The family was elated when a marriage proposal came from the neighbouring textile town of Ichalkaranji. The boy was a booking clerk at a cinema hall and his family had farmland as well. Sunanda's father was so happy that he decided that the marriage should take place immediately. Young Sunanda was unable to understand why a boy from a comparatively well-off family was ready to marry her. She tried to speak to her father and asked him to check the boy's background. But her father refused to do so, saying that there was no need to enquire about the boy and his family.

Once married, Sunanda was pushed into motherhood. She delivered a weak baby boy who frequently fell ill. Soon, Sunanda realised that something was wrong with her as well. She felt fatigued and gasped for breath all the time. Her husband took her to the local doctor, who gave Sunanda and the baby some pills. However, their illness grew worse and the baby expired eight months after birth. Sunanda was unable to understand what was happening. But there were more shocks waiting for her. Her husband, who was coughing frequently, was diagnosed with TB.

'That day, my in-laws kicked us out of the house.

We were left with no option but to live in a cattle shed near the house. Over the next few days, my husband was completely paralysed and unable to move. He stopped working and now, we had nothing to eat. We were starving in the cattle shed,' recalls Sunanda. School children in the locality noticed their plight and gave their pocket money to the couple. Some boys from the area went shopping and bought them food. When Sunanda's family members came to know about this they scolded the boys and told their parents to keep their kids away from Sunanda and her husband.

But some women in the locality, realising that Sunanda and her husband were deteriorating, came to their aid. 'When these women came to meet us, our family members warned them. But some of the women continued to support us and came with rotis, which they hid in their blouses. We ate everything that we could during those days,' says Sunanda. Her husband was not getting the needed treatment for TB. 'People told me that TB is curable and I wanted to treat him. But somehow, he was not willing to be treated,' says Sunanda.

One day, while Sunanda was sitting in the cattle shed, her husband walked in and fell at her feet. She did not understand why or what he was doing. He broke down and overcome with emotion, was unable to speak. Eventually, when he spoke, Sunanda froze. There was complete darkness before her and she nearly collapsed. 'Please forgive me...forgive me,' he pleaded. He confessed that he was a frequent visitor to the redlight area in the city and was an HIV patient. It was detected when he went to donate blood at a blood donation camp. But he had never revealed any of this to Sunanda. The man died a few days later, leaving Sunanda with nothing but an HIV infection. Sunanda felt deceived, but nobody was willing to help her.

Finding Inner Strength

With the death of Sunanda's husband, her in-laws wanted her to leave the cattle shed and the town immediately. They told her that they had nothing to do with her after the death of their son. Baffled by what was happening, Sunanda, who had no other place to go, went back to her parents. Her father was unwilling to take her back, but her mother opened the doors of the family home to her. Her parents went to Sunanda's in-laws to discuss her future, but they were told that the matter had already ended.

'We have lost gold (their son) and what will we do with this deadwood (Sunanda)?' they said. It was clear that the in-laws wanted to completely cut off Sunanda to discourage her from making any claim on the family property. 'She is not our responsibility and because of her our son got an HIV infection and TB,' they alleged.

With her education incomplete, and laid low by various health issues, Sunanda was in a quagmire. Her father worried that having a widowed daughter with the HIV 'stigma' would create problems for their family. He was more anxious about his younger son and his future. Except for her mother, nobody wanted Sunanda around. She sank into depression and thought of ending her life. 'I asked myself why I should live and for whom,' she recalls.

'I don't know exactly, but while thinking about ending my life, I also started wondering why I had to suffer and die when I had not committed any mistake. In our society, the majority of women are deprived of their rights and suffer silently. I felt agitated and angry. By ending my life what would change? Nothing. But if I put up a fight for my rights, at least I would get the satisfaction of not succumbing to injustice,' she says.

Sunanda started to work in the silver industry while being treated for HIV. She enrolled in a junior college to complete her twelfth standard. Her neighbours ridiculed her saying that she was going to spread HIV among the college students. At that time, she also approached a sessions court to lay claim to her husband's share of the family property.

Amidst all this came another twist in her journey.

Spinal Challenge

Sunanda continued fighting battles on multiple fronts. But all of a sudden, she started facing problems walking and just standing up straight. She went to an orthopedic doctor, who treated her. But the pain did not subside. 'I was finding it difficult to breathe. I tried various treatments as no one was able to diagnose what had happened,' she says. Sunanda continued to receive different treatments for back pain and breathlessness. Later, an MRI of the spine at a private hospital in Karad in Satara district would reveal that she had spinal TB.

The 'Index—TB guidelines on extra-pulmonary TB for India' state that all patients with suspected TB of the spine require an MRI to assess the extent of the disease and the degree of bone destruction. It is also necessary to confirm spinal cord involvement in patients with neurological signs. An MRI is useful in making a diagnosis in the early stages of the disease, while some MRI images clearly indicate a diagnosis of spinal TB.

It was already too late for Sunanda by the time she was diagnosed with spinal TB. The Index TB guidelines highlight that a TB infection of the bones and joints causes chronic pain, deformity, and disability while cervical spine TB can be life-threatening. Bone and joint TB makes up about 10%

of this type of TB. Spinal TB is the most common form of TB, both children and adults can suffer from it. This kind of TB, where localised back pain can continue for more than six weeks, is disabling. Advanced-stage patients face severe pain and spinal deformities along with paraspinal muscle wasting and a neurological deficit. Children who suffer because of this TB will face additional issues. They fail to thrive, suffer night cries (in their sleep) and are also unable to walk, or walk with a cautious gait, using their hands to support the head or trunk, according to the guidelines, which are an initiative of the Central TB Division, Ministry of Health and Family Welfare, Government of India.[1]

'Finally, I went to the government hospital, where doctors gave me tablets. I was told there that I had water in my spine, and by this time I was not able to stand even for a few minutes,' says Sunanda. The doctors at the government hospital told her that spinal TB is not easily curable. As the pain became unbearable, she requested the doctors to change her treatment, but they said that the pain would lessen with time. She wanted to be treated by private doctors but had no money for this. An X-ray of the chest, HIV test, X-ray of the spine, MRI of the spine, CT spine, and biopsy of the lesion is used to reach a diagnosis. But basic health infrastructure still remains out of the reach of the economically backward like Sunanda.

Pathetic Health Infrastructure

An increase in public spending on healthcare can significantly reduce Out of Pocket Expenditure (OOPE) from 65% to 35% of the overall healthcare spend and reduce the financial burden of patients like Sunanda. India has one of the highest levels of OOPE in the world. This adds directly to the high incidence of catastrophic expenditure and poverty. Patients like Sunanda have to face a double challenge: suffer because of a late diagnosis and remain deprived of quality treatment because of the lack of money. India's public health expenditure stood between 1.2% to 1.6% of GDP between 2008-09 and 2019-20. The Economic Survey 2020-21 recommended an increase in public spending on healthcare services from 1% to 2.5-3% of the GDP. The existing expenditure is relatively low as compared to other countries such as China (3.2%), the US (8.5%), and Germany (9.4%) according to PRS Legislative Research.[2]

A NITI Aayog study on the 'not-for-profit hospital' model in India states that India has achieved economic growth and modernisation but unavailability and unaffordability of healthcare services remain a major challenge. India has a lower bed density (number of hospital beds per 1,000 population) than the rest of the world. The bed density in India is 1.0, in low-income countries it is 1.2, in middle-income countries it is 2.4, and worldwide it is 2.7.[3]

Availability of beds and hospitals in India is concentrated in urban areas. This has a direct impact on accessibility and affordability of hospitalisation services. Overall, 72% of hospital beds in India are in urban areas while just 28% are in rural areas.[4]

The allopathic doctor-population ratio in India is 1:1,404, per the current population estimate of 1.35 billion. This is well below the WHO norm of 1:1,000. Interestingly, 52% of these doctors practise in just five States: Maharashtra, Tamil Nadu, Karnataka, Andhra Pradesh (and Telangana), and Uttar Pradesh.

The Will to Survive

Optimum management of spinal TB requires the involvement of multiple specialists, including a spinal orthopedic surgeon, microbiologist/infectious diseases specialist and spinal radiologist, as well as physiotherapists and orthotists. All presumptive spinal TB cases should be referred to and managed in specialist centres, according to the recommendations of the index TB guidelines on extra-pulmonary TB.

The lack of expert doctors and proper treatment in the government system forced Sunanda to seek private treatment. She was admitted to a private Trust Hospital at Panchgani in Satara. The treatment continued for one-and–a-half years. Sunanda says that the delay in diagnosis and proper treatment affected her spinal cord. She recovered to a good extent but suffers spinal pain once in a while even today.

'Already, I was facing discrimination because of HIV, and TB added to the pain and insults. Even my closest relatives were unwilling to talk to me. But my mother, who is just a fourth-standard pass, stood firmly with me,' says Sunanda.

While fighting TB and HIV, Sunanda continued her battle in the courts. Her in-laws told the court that their son had no HIV infection and that Sunanda was lying. Sunanda staked her savings on a court case and won the battle at the sessions court. Her in-laws went to the district court and then to the High Court. But the High Court refused to hear the case and asked her in-laws to give Sunanda her share of the property. Sunanda approached her in-laws to take control of a half-acre of land and a room allocated by the court as her share of the property. They locked the room and refused to give away the farmland. Sunanda went to the police. When she got control of the property, she decided to sell it, but her in-laws created all kinds of hurdles to prevent a deal from going through.

Amidst all these difficulties, Sunanda completed her graduation in Arts and Masters in Sociology and the Marathi language. She wanted to become a teacher by pursuing a diploma in Elementary Education. But she decided to pay donations for her brother so that he could complete his education. 'See the irony of life. I educated my brother, but the same brother spat on my face one day saying that I have brought disgrace upon the family. I decided to step out of the house and be on my own. I joined an NGO and then joined as a coordinator at the antiretroviral therapy (ART) department at the government hospital in Kolhapur,' says Sunanda.

While working as a coordinator, Sunanda also developed a matrimonial app to connect HIV-infected people who want to marry. She herself married an HIV-infected person a few years ago. 'I have arranged dozens of marriages of HIV-infected people. We have every right to live. Believe me, the majority of women who come to us are deprived and deceived. They get infected by men and are deserted,' says Sunanda.

*

It is late in the evening in Kolhapur and the skies are clear. The man and the woman sitting in front of Sunanda are smiling broadly. They have decided to grow a spine. Sunanda's life has become a guiding light for HIV and TB patients in the region.

I asked Sunanda if I could use her name and her picture in this book.

'Of course, you can. I have announced it myself and told my story in public with my name. Also, I have nothing to hide. What is there to hide in HIV and TB?' she asks. 'Write my name as Sunanda alias Rupali. Many people know me by either of these names,' she says, happily posing for a picture.

'Please write that HIV and TB are not the end of the world,' she tells me with admirable confidence.

NOTES

1. World Health Organization. Country Office for India. (2016). Index-TB guidelines: guidelines on extra-pulmonary tuberculosis in India. Retrieved from https://apps.who.int/iris/handle/10665/278953
2. PRS Legislative Research. (no date). Demand for Grants 2020-21 Analysis: Health and Family Welfare. Retrieved from https://prsindia.org/budgets/parliament/demand-for-grants-2020-21-analysis-health-and-family-welfare
3. NITI Aayog. (2021) Study on Not for Profit Hospital Model in India. Retrieved from https://www.niti.gov.in/node/1543
4. PTI. (2013). Study reveals rural India gets only 1/3rd of hospital beds. Retrieved from https://www.thehindu.com/sci-tech/health/study-reveals-rural-india-gets-only-13rd-of-hospital-beds/article4931844.ece

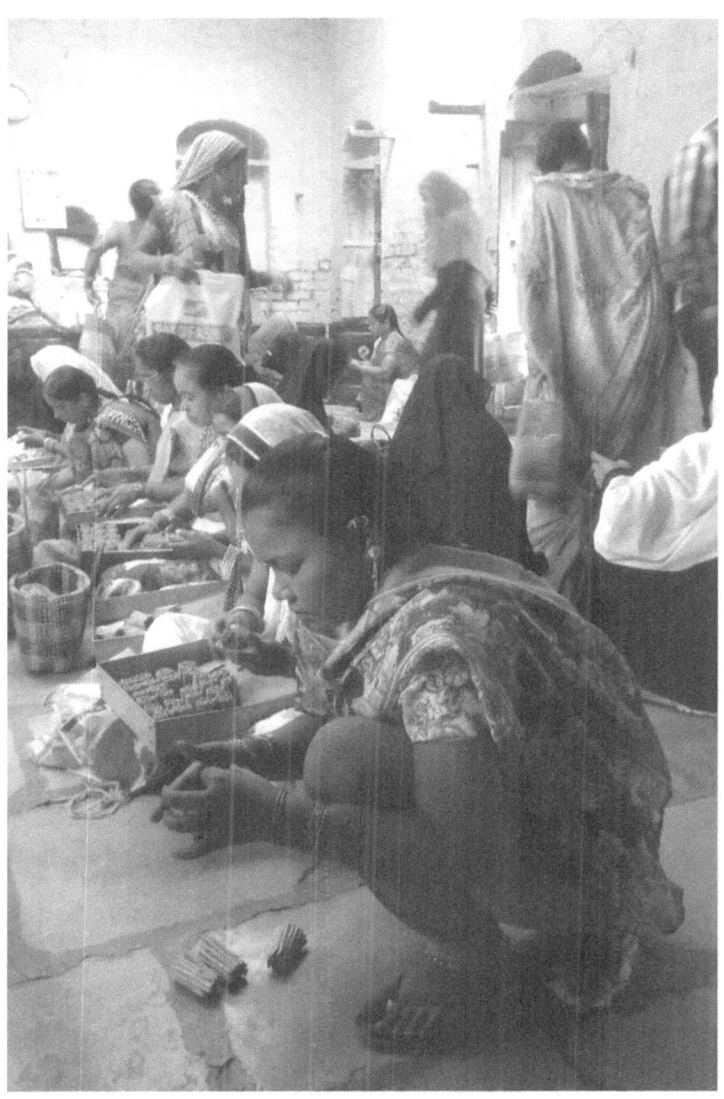

Solapur's bidi rollers are stuck in a dilemma. They know what is ailing them, but they cannot acknowledge it openly or seek treatment. *(picture credit: Suryakant Asbe)*

4

Livelihood and TB: Rolling Death

It is late afternoon and the bidi-roller women in Solapur's Duttanagar slums are speeding up their work. They will not get a tea break today as there are many bidis to be rolled and deposited in the bidi factory for packing.

Solapur is famed throughout India as a textile town. What is less known is that it is also Maharashtra's bidi capital. Bidis are small cigarettes—essentially tobacco flakes hand-rolled in tendu leaves. And while tobacco in all its forms—be it cigarettes, cigars, bidis or gutka, has been scientifically proven to be harmful to human life, for the women of Solapur, it is something that supports life and sustains it.

The bidi-rolling women sit around winnowing baskets filled with tendu leaves. Close at hand are tobacco flakes, scissors, and a thread bundle. They pick up a leaf, cut it into shape, place a pinch of tobacco on it, and dexterously roll the leaf into a bidi without breaking it. Lastly, they tie the bidi with a roll of thread and toss it into an aluminium tray before starting on the next one. The entire process takes just a few seconds. Within a few minutes there are dozens of bidis in the aluminium tray.

As the women continue rolling bidis in one of the houses in the slum, two girls in school outfits watch them with rapt attention. Outside, there are 4-5 groups of drunk men busy playing cards under a tree.

While rolling the bidis a woman croons in Telugu. When asked what the song is about, she just smiles and stops crooning. After a few moments of silence, she explains that it is a dialogue between a mother and her child. 'In the song, the mother is talking about her dreams for the child. In fact, all mothers dream for their children,' says another woman, who translates her Telugu counterpart's explanation into Hindi.

As they converse, the women continue to work mechanically. Bidi rolling is manual at all stages, but these women perform the task like machines. For over a century, women in Solapur have rolled bidis, with the older ones training the next generation to continue the tradition. For generations, families from parts of Andhra Pradesh and Telangana have settled in Solapur and the majority of the Telugu women are into bidi rolling.

'This is the life skill we teach our girls. Once they have this skill, life becomes easier,' says an old woman in the group, flashing a tattered yellow card. 'This is our credit card, our Aadhar card, which supports our living,' she declares. The other women nod in agreement. 'Once our girls have this card, there is no need for a college certificate or degree. Girls who have this card are in demand in the marriage market and parents don't have to pay a dowry,' the old woman explains.

Nineteen-year-old Radha Dhanewale knows the importance of the card. She is one of the lucky girls who has earned this card. Not surprisingly, she is a sought-after bride in the community. A resident of the congested Lodhi lane in a town dominated by poor labourers, Radha, like many other girls, left school to learn bidi rolling.

'I learned the skill from my mother. I used to skip classes and my mother allowed me to do so only if I agreed to learn bidi rolling. School education would not have fetched me a job, but my bidi-rolling skills have paid off. I got a bidi card a few years ago and now my life is settled. I don't have to worry much about marriage nor will my family have to think of dowry,' says Radha. 'Getting a bidi card is like having a government job.' Many girls like her are putting in an effort into honing their skills rolling bidis so that they, too, get the card and are set for life.

The bidi card is a piece of paper issued by bidi factories to skilled women. It assures them of bidi-rolling work for a lifetime, along with other benefits such as provident fund, bonus, and medical help. The daily output of the women workers is registered on these cards. But the cards are given only to women who are highly skilled.

While the men were losing their jobs in the textile sector, the women in Solapur were rolling bidis for about 200 branded bidi factories across the country. The women held the fort for their families during the Covid-19 crisis, thanks to the bidi cards. These cards helped them sustain their families and raise money from formal and informal lenders in Solapur.

'I roll about 1,000 bidis every day and earn Rs 140 daily. My company also deducts my provident fund contribution from my earnings. If I need more money, I roll more bidis. Also, I don't have to step out of the house for work. I roll bidis at home and deposit the bundles at the end of the day in the factory,' Radha adds. Many men who do not allow women to step out of the home for work are happy with the bidi work as it is considered 'safe for women'. Women have to visit the bidi factory only to collect raw material and deposit the bidis.

They roll bidis for about 7-8 hours at home while taking care of daily chores. This makes bidi rolling the favourite employment for women in the town.

Twenty-one-year-old Priyanka insists that every girl wants to study and complete her education. 'But you see what is happening around. Those who have degrees have no jobs. I liked my school, but along with studies, I learned to roll bidis,' she says. A resident of Kuchannagar, Priyanka discontinued her studies after the twelfth standard and is happily married. 'The bidi card has made life happier and easier. When you don't have any other option, you select what is available,' she adds. In fact, these bidi-roller women are the main earners in hundreds of households in the city's slums.

'Many of them (men) have no jobs. The city's economy largely runs around textiles and bidis. Besides over 50,000 bidi rollers, about 10,000 people directly and indirectly depend on the bidi industry. Solapur has the highest number of sugar factories in the State and the textile industry is still active. But there is no employment for women in these sectors. In fact, there are limited job opportunities as the industrial sector is on its deathbed,' says Communist Party of India (Marxist) leader and former MLA Narsayya Adam. He adds that the government has frequently made announcements that women should stop rolling bidis as it is hazardous to the health of smokers.

'Why just smokers? Even bidi rollers suffer heavily due to this work. These poor women have to pay the heavy cost of earning a livelihood by rolling bidis. As a child, I saw my mother coughing blood. She rolled bidis day and night. She had TB and died in 1985 without much medical help. Our poverty proved fatal,' says an emotional Adam (75), who is popularly known as Adam Master. 'Women here don't roll bidis because they like it; they do it because they don't have any option but to cling to those bidi cards,' he adds.

A Card with a Heavy Price

But this 'credit card' comes at a cost. Some of the health effects experienced by bidi workers include pain and cramps in the shoulders, neck, back, and lower abdomen. The incidence of tuberculosis and bronchial asthma is higher than it is among the general population, according to research by the Factory Advisory Services and Labour Institute in Bombay, a unit of the Labour Ministry of India. The 'Bidi Smoking and Public Health' report published in 2008 by the Ministry of Health and Family Welfare, in partnership with the WHO, adds that since the 1970s, trade union leaders had expressed their concerns that 50% of bidi workers eventually die from tuberculosis or asthma. Bidi workers work in congested houses without ventilation and TB can be easily transmitted in these smoky homes, which use brick or mud chulhas (stoves) for cooking. Bidi workers are exposed to tobacco dust and indoor pollution.

The report also highlights the association between TB and poor nutrition. Bidi rollers complain of loss of appetite because of the smell of their raw material. 'Bidi workers recognise the negative health effects and some women attempt to reduce the harm by drinking small amounts of nutritional supplements (tonic) or taking multi-vitamin injections, a popular practice in some areas of South India,' the report adds.[1]

The International Labour Organization (ILO) Note on India's bidi sector lists the common ailments suffered by bidi-rolling women. They include postural problems (neck and lower back pain), abdominal pain, eye problems, a burning sensation in the throat, cough, asthma, tuberculosis, bronchitis, excessive bleeding during menstruation, irregular and painful menstrual cycles, leucorrhea, anemia, anemic body aches, and dizziness from constant exposure to tobacco dust.[2]

When I ask the group of women rolling bidis in the Duttanagar slums about TB and other occupational health problems, I am met with pindrop silence. The women refuse to make eye contact and answer questions. After some prodding, one of them replies, saying, 'You tell us what to do. Should we die without food?' Women here feel that anyone who questions their bidi rolling is from the government or anti-tobacco campaign teams and wants to snatch away their work.

Sitting in the dingy, congested shanties these women breathe tobacco dust every day and are very aware of TB. They have seen many TB cases around but do not want to discuss the disease.

'Yes. There are TB cases, but don't relate everything to bidi rolling. We will stop bidi rolling the day government officers find us alternative work. If you care so much about us, give us jobs. If you think that we will die because of TB, remember that if you stop our work we will die of hunger. Nobody talks about cigarettes as it is an addiction of rich people and the production is by big companies. Everyone wants to target the poor,' says one woman. The others in the damp room nod in agreement.

Local scribe Suryakant Asbe, who has studied bidi workers for years, says that life is a vicious cycle for them. 'In recent times, there has been a lot of pressure from various groups and even from the government that bidis should be banned. It is a fact that smoking is injurious to health, but it is also injurious to bidi rollers. Many bidi rollers don't even get basic treatment for TB. The majority don't even realise that they have TB and keep taking some other medicines.' Asbe adds that life in the slums has been unhealthy for decades.

When women talk about TB, they want to insist that it is not a 'big problem'. They fear that if TB in the city is highlighted in the media, NGOs and the government will get another reason to impose a ban on bidis.

Fight for Rights

Though they are not willing to admit it, the women know that this hazardous work is taking a toll on their health. 'Men are unwilling to spend on the health of the women who earn money. We are just money-making machines who have to die rolling bidis,' says Yellama. Like the others, she insists that bidi rolling and smoking have nothing to do with TB or cancer and adds that spending even Rs 10 to buy tablets disturbs their monthly budget. The majority of households in economically backward localities depend on a monthly income of about Rs 3,000-4,000 earned by the bidi-rolling women. The men earn money sometimes, but spend the majority of their earnings on liquor. Fear of medical expenditure keeps most of the bidi-roller women away from hospitals.

Not surprisingly, the 2020-21 Economic Survey notes that India has one of the highest levels of OOPE in the world. A negative correlation exists between the level of public spending and OOPE both across countries and States.[3]

The 'Tracking Universal Health Coverage: 2017 Global Monitoring Report' by the World Bank and the World Health Organization reveals that 800 million people spend at least 10% of their household budgets on health expenditure on themselves, a sick child, or other family members. The report states that 4.16% and 4.61% of households in India, based on two different poverty lines, are forced for impoverishing spending on health.[4]

Stigma, poverty, and the fear of losing work keeps women away from getting themselves checked for TB. The bidi rollers already have a lot on their plate, fighting for the basics. They have to fight against poverty, male-dominated families and society, the government's obsolete mechanisms, and ruthless politicians. The fight is also against themselves. Solapur's bidi rollers are stuck in a dilemma. They know what is ailing them, but cannot acknowledge it openly or seek treatment.

Many women feel that if they go to a hospital for TB or cancer treatment, it would threaten their livelihood. The general consensus is that whatever happens to individuals, their livelihood must not be affected.

The WHO insists that community engagement has a big role to play in TB prevention, diagnosis, and treatment, especially where people with TB have poor access to formal health services. Community engagement for TB covers a wide range of activities for the identification, referral, and treatment of people with drug-susceptible, drug-resistant, and HIV-associated TB.[5] But when the community itself is in denial, community engagement becomes a major challenge.

The Future of Bidi Rollers' Betis

The Central government is implementing the Prime Minister's ambitious Beti Bachao, Beti Padhao (BBBP) scheme in Solapur. The scheme aims to address the declining Child Sex Ratio (CSR) and lack of empowerment of girls and women over a lifecycle continuum.[6]

For the betis (daughters) of bidi rollers in Solapur, life is far from positive. Their future is still lost and invisible in the tobacco dust all around them. 'Do you think that we don't want to see our children becoming a collector (district magistrate) or a doctor? Do you think we want to continue in hazardous working conditions?' asks sixty-year-old Nalini Kalburgi, who works with unorganized sector workers. She says that bidi-rolling women want their future generations to live a healthy life, but admits that the fear of losing a livelihood is much bigger than the fear of contracting TB.

'If bidi rolling is snatched away from these women,

they will commit suicide or consume poison. What else can they do? Those who blame us should provide us employment. And anyway, we are not sitting idle. Women are trying every possible way to build a better life for themselves and to secure the future of their children,' Kalburgi adds.

After fighting a legal battle for years, bidi workers have earned rights as industrial employees and receive all the benefits employees are entitled to under various government acts. In 2006, after a long, collective effort, 10,000 low-cost houses for women bidi workers were completed and inaugurated under the Comrade Godutai Parulekar Housing Scheme. The houses were built with equal contributions from the workers and from the State and Central governments. In 2015, a smaller programme with 1,600 similar houses for women bidi workers, called the Comrade Meenakshitai Sane Housing Scheme, was inaugurated. Another 30,000 homes are being built in Kumbhari village on the outskirts of Solapur for unorganized sector workers, mainly bidi and textile workers.

The dream of good housing is coming true after decades of struggle. Kalburgi says that the new houses will create livable conditions with good ventilation. 'This will also help reduce population density. The new houses are much better than the slums. This is a small beginning towards a change. Any change cannot be forced. We are trying to get the new generation out of the bidi world,' she adds.

NOTES

1. Gupta, P. & Asma S. (Ed.). (2008). Bidi Smoking and Public Health. Retrieved from https://www.who.int/tobacco/publications/prod_regulation/bidi_smoking_public_health.pdf
2. International Labour Organization (2003). Bidi Sector in India: A Note. Retrieved from https://www.ilo.org/wcmsp5/groups/public/—asia/—ro-bangkok/—sro-new_delhi/documents/projectdocumentation/wcms_125466.pdf
3. Ministry of Finance, Government of India (2020-21). Economic Survey. Retrieved from https://www.indiabudget.gov.in/economicsurvey/
4. World Health Organization, The World Bank (2017). Tracking Universal Health Coverage: 2017 Global Monitoring Report. Retrieved from https://apps.who.int/iris/bitstream/handle/10665/259817/9789241513555-eng.pdf
5. World Health Organization (2015). Empowering Communities to End TB with the Engage TB approach. Retrieved from https://www.who.int/tb/areas-of-work/community-engagement/ENGAGE_TB_Brochure.pdf?ua=1
6. Lok Sabha (2021). Unstarred Question No 897. Retrieved from http://164.100.24.220/loksabhaquestions/annex/176/AU897.pdf

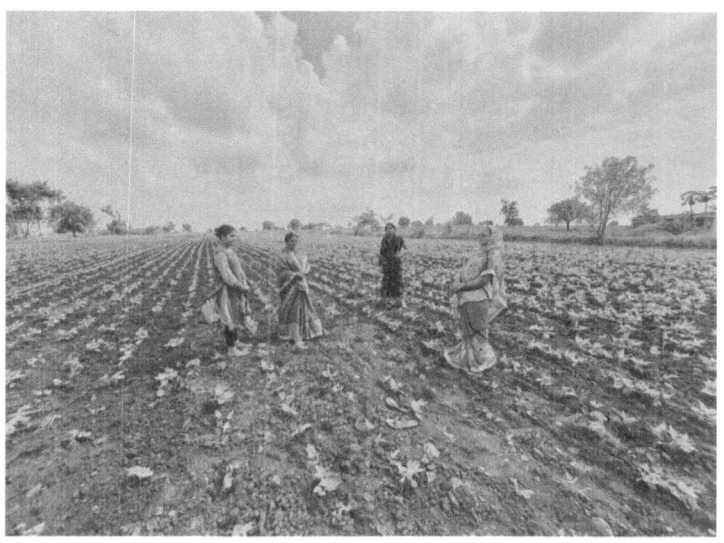

Single women, widows, and abandoned women are easy prey. 'Others will not understand what a single woman has to go through,' says Sunanda Kharate (seen right in pic).
(picture credit: Radheshyam Jadhav)

5

Abandoned Women and TB: A Lonely Battle

Nanda's (name changed) husband considered it normal to thrash her repeatedly. She, too, accepted the beatings as a part of life. Indeed, for a long time, she did not consider it to be domestic violence, and viewed it as her husband's right. Nanda suffered immense mental and physical trauma. She had a chronic cough and was not getting proper treatment for it. Her husband was agitated about having to give her money every time she went to the hospital. Depressed, Nanda finally decided to leave her husband.

She had nowhere to go. Like many other families in India, Nanda's parents proudly believed that a woman must see sunlight only twice in her lifetime.

First, when she is married and crosses the threshold of her father's house to enter her husband's house, and second, when her dead body is carried out of her husband's house. Not surprisingly, Nanda decided not to return to her parental house or to any other relatives.

Nanda had never imagined that she would one day leave her husband's house. But she was left with no other option as she could not cope with the torture. She is not alone. The National Family Health Survey 4 (NFHS 4) has recorded that gender-based violence against women has been acknowledged worldwide as a violation of basic human rights. Research shows that such violence results in health burdens, intergenerational effects, and demographic consequences. As per the survey, 33% of married women have experienced physical, sexual, or emotional spousal violence. 'The most common type of spousal violence is physical violence (30%), followed by emotional violence (14%). 7% of married women have experienced spousal sexual violence,' according to the survey. Interestingly, 52% of women and 42% of men believe that a husband is justified in beating his wife in at least one of seven specified circumstances: when she goes out without informing him, neglects the house or the children, argues with him, refuses to have sex with him, doesn't cook food properly, suspects her of being unfaithful, and when she is disrespectful to her in-laws. Only 14% of women who have experienced physical or sexual violence by anyone have sought help to stop the violence.[1]

Nanda is among the huge majority of women who had no support and help to stop the violence. She reached Ichalkaranji (Kolhapur district) bus stop and was at a crossroads, unsure about which way to turn. Her cough was bothering her and she suspected TB. All these months she had wanted to tell her husband that she needed a TB a check-up. But her husband was already unhappy over spending money on her health problems.

The National Framework for a Gender-Responsive Approach to TB in India, published by the Central TB Division, Ministry of Health and Family Welfare, notes that studies indicate that there are various reasons for the reporting of fewer cases of TB among women. These include poor access to healthcare services, poor diagnosis, and poor reporting of cases among women. 'Multiple studies on the incidence of TB, across the country, indicate that more men report microbiologically confirmed pulmonary TB, and women are more likely to have clinically diagnosed pulmonary TB and extra-pulmonary forms of TB,' the report states. It also adds that there is evidence that presentation of pulmonary TB among women may be different from men. This contributes to delays and makes it difficult to diagnose TB in women. 'While men generally present with fever, hemoptysis, and night sweats, women could present with common symptoms or non-specific findings such as fever, body ache, loss of appetite, and fatigue,' the report adds.[2]

Life Trial

Nanda's cough was getting worse by the day. 'An abandoned woman is probably the most helpless and vulnerable human being. She is vulnerable to all types of exploitation,' says Anuradha Bhosale of the Kolhapur-based Ekati organization, which works for abandoned women.

When Nanda reached Ekati with the help of civic workers, she was devastated and unwilling to live. What she had experienced after leaving her home was horrible. She was taken to a hospital and the doctors found that she had asthma, not TB. When she came to know that she was not a TB patient, she saw a ray of hope. As she was trying to stand on her own, her husband came to take her back. Forgetting the past, Nanda happily returned with him. After all, he was her 'pati parmeshwar'—her saviour and protector. She was happy to be home even though she was not sure how her husband was going to treat her.

'It's a choice between a brick and a stone for

women. Many women face all kinds of exploitation at their husband's house and want to leave him, but they don't have any other option. In rural areas, you will find that the majority of women are not educated and fear that if they leave their husband's house, society will target them in all kinds of ways. Men are like vultures. Single women, a widow or an abandoned woman are easy prey. You won't understand what a single woman has to go through. And because of this the majority of women tolerate torture, and stay with their husbands,' says Sunanda Kharate, who herself is a single woman living in Osmanabad district of Maharashtra. Sunanda is a feisty feminist who locked horns with society and continues to live alone. She joined the NGO working for women and farmers, and actively helps others today.

But Shanta (name changed) was not fortunate enough to meet someone like Sunanda. At the age of 65, she was kicked out of the house by her son and daughter-in-law. Suffering from pulmonary TB, she reached the famous Mahalaxmi temple in Kolhapur and started begging. She was lying on the roadside and was taken to the government hospital by civic workers. Tests revealed that she had TB and the hospital authorities, with the help of the NGO, started looking for her relatives. Shanta herself was not able to recall anything and likely did not want to return home. Her TB treatment continued for four months but she was then diagnosed with breast cancer. As nobody was bothered about her, the treatment she received was intermittent. Finally, she succumbed to cancer.

Genital TB and Fertility

Shanta could at least talk about her TB, which is not the case with those who have genital TB. A report titled 'A Rapid Assessment of Gender and Tuberculosis in India' jointly published by REACH, Stop TB Partnership, and UNOPS in 2018, states that genital TB is an under-diagnosed and neglected form of TB among women. Using various references and studies, the report states that genital TB generally affects the fallopian tubes, endometrium, and ovaries and is recognised to be a leading cause of infertility among women. 'Figures from India indicate that 9% of all extra-pulmonary TB cases are genital TB. An ICMR paper has noted an increase in the prevalence of female genital TB in women seeking treatment for infertility from 19% in 2011 to 30% in 2015,' the report states. A systematic review and meta-analysis of existing studies shows that nearly 24% of all cases of infertility are estimated to be on account of TB. Genital TB is generally silent (shows no symptoms for a long time) and difficult to diagnose, the report adds.

Genital TB is silent in most cases and is discovered during the work-up to diagnose the causes of infertility. Some women experience reduced menstruation, amenorrhea or irregular menstrual cycles. Others have vaginal discharge and abdominal pain. TB in such conditions can be treated, but there is a possibility of the fallopian tubes or endometrium getting damaged in the process to regain fertility. There is also a high possibility of ectopic pregnancies (outside the uterus) and miscarriages. The report highlights that in a country like India, where getting married and bearing children is the norm, infertility causes significant emotional trauma to the woman and often invites harassment and discrimination. In a patriarchal society, women having a male child get acceptance and respect. 'Childless women, therefore, often live in perpetual insecurity of being deserted or of the husband taking a second wife. Infertile women are often not invited to religious ceremonies or may be excluded from some rituals in social events, making their sense of discrimination acute,' the report adds.[3]

'There are very few female doctors, medical supervisors, and health workers in the government set-up. TB is taboo and talking about genital TB is impossible. When a widow or abandoned woman comes forward with problems, she is not sure how she will be treated and in what way she will be exploited,' admits a medical officer working in the Government of Maharashtra's TB section.

Controlling the Power

TB diagnosis and treatment is a distant dream for women in the remote Lasina village in Maharashtra's Yavatmal district. Yet, these rural women have made a small but confident beginning when it comes to managing their health. They have started using sanitary napkins. This might sound trivial, but it is a major development for women in the area. A few years ago, women in Lasina also established a strong network of self-help groups and started small ventures like poultry, goat rearing, and shops.

Women are saving up money to address their own health issues. Geetmala Bhandare explains that agrarian distress is perennial in the region and poverty and losses in agriculture have a direct impact on health expenditure. Men continue to drink and smoke even when there is nothing to eat in the house. But if a woman is unwell, she is not allowed to go to the hospital. 'Sanitary pads were considered a fad of city women. We continue to use unhygienic methods of menstrual protection, mostly cloth and sometimes, ashes and husk,' she says. This could lead to bacteria infecting the urinary tract or the uterus.

As the women started to save money, they began

to use sanitary napkins. Alka Kamble, a local woman who was the sarpanch of the village and has political ambitions, says health issues like TB and cancer can have cascading effects on the lives of women. 'You can understand the situation. If there is no money to buy a sanitary napkin, how can you even think of treating big diseases?' she asks. Alka has the answer to her own question. 'Women should work and not depend on their husbands. That's why we started self-help groups. Now, we have some money so, we can pay attention to our health. See, bhau (brother), you must have the power to live with dignity. I am not talking about political power, but control of land, money, and your work. Only then will you be able to control your own life,' she says.

Women do not have much faith in government health services as they say that the economically backward are neglected in government hospitals. At the same time, they cannot afford private treatment, and depend on inadequate government services.

Meanwhile, women who joined hands to resist the violence of their husbands and formed organizations have taken up more empowerment agendas. One such experiment was started in Uttar Pradesh. The Gulabi Gang movement was started in 2006 by Sampat Pal Devi in Banda district, which is one of the poorest districts in the country, and dominated by patriarchal culture and domestic violence. The new Green Gang movement in Varanasi's villages is fighting against drug and liquor consumption along with domestic violence with the help of youth. 'It is a movement by women to protect their own rights and also to develop villages,' says activist Ravi Mishra, who supports these women in Khusiyari village.

NOTES

1. Ministry of Health and Family Welfare. (2015-16). National Family Health Survey 2015-16. Retrieved from http://rchiips.org/nfhs/nfhs-4Reports/India.pdf
2. Central TB Division, Ministry of Health and Family Welfare. (2019). National Framework for a Gender-responsive approach to TB in India. Retrieved from—https://tbcindia.gov.in/WriteReadData/l892s/388838054811%20NTEP%20Gender%20Responsive%20Framework_311219.pdf
3. REACH, Stop TB Partnership, and UNOPS. (2018). A Rapid Assessment of Gender and Tuberculosis in India. Retrieved from http://www.stoptb.org/assets/documents/communities/CRG/TB%20Gender%20Assessment%20India.pdf

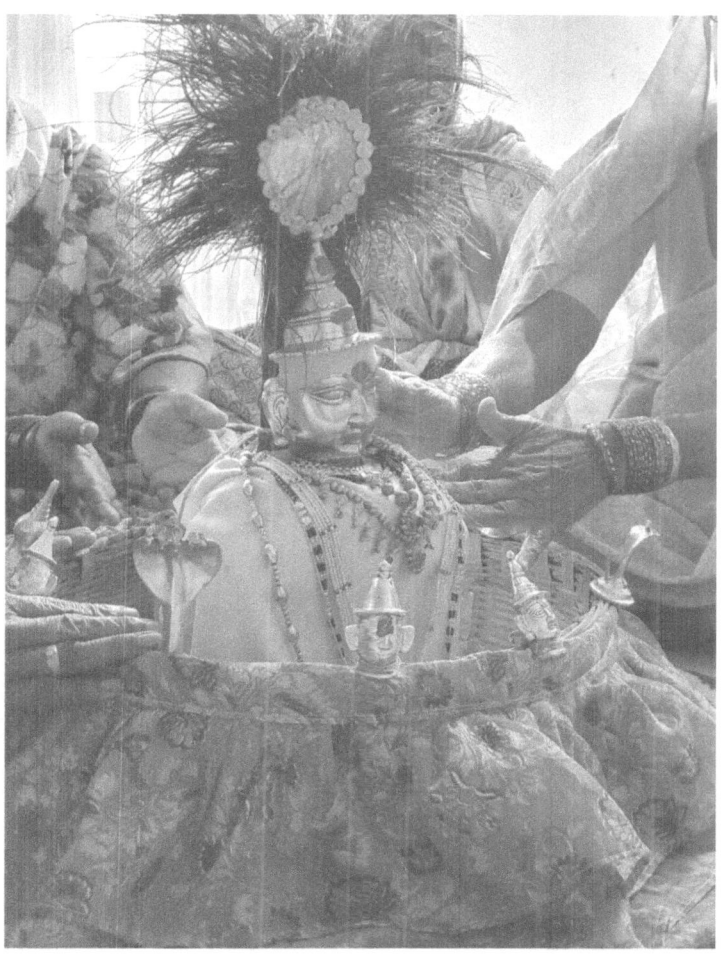

Goddess Yellamma: Why do hundreds of devadasis die of AIDS, TB, and other diseases without treatment? Devadasis look in vain to Goddess Yellamma to answer their question.
(picture credit: Radheshyam Jadhav)

6

Faith and TB: God's Curse

'Awwa, ninde seve madak bandina' (Mother, I am coming to serve you), sings septuagenarian Sushila, praising Goddess Yellamma in Kannada in a trembling voice as she decorates the mukhota (brass image of Goddess Yellamma's face). She ensures that the vermilion on the forehead of the Goddess is smeared accurately.

As she folds her hands and closes her eyes, other women sitting around imitate her. 'Aai (Mother), save your children from this Covid. You have saved us from all diseases and problems. Because of you, we are safe,' she says, keeping the mask she had worn until now aside. The other women do the same.

Sushila is a devadasi. She is also the leader of the devadasis in the Kolhapur-Nipani region. Everyone from the local MLA, who is a minister in the State cabinet, to the village leaders, knows Sushila well. She has spent her entire life in this region bordering Karnataka and Maharashtra.

It is 9.30 a.m. and Sushila, who belongs to Nipani in Karnataka, has settled into her house in Annbhau Sathe Nagar, in the town of Kagal, Kolhapur district. 'There is nothing to do. Our Mother's house (temple) is closed because of this Covid. Otherwise, our day starts early. We take jag (round basket made of bamboo strips in which a brass image of Yellamma is kept) house-to-house, seeking jogva (alms). But for the last one-and-a-half years everything is at a standstill. The government must help us,' she says. The other women murmur in agreement.

'So, you have come to enquire about TB patients among devadasis?' she asks me.

'Yes. Yesterday, you said you would connect me to a TB patient,' I say.

Now, there is complete silence in the room. Sushila is trying to frame her response.

'There are some cases here and there, but we don't face any major problem. Rather, we don't have many devadasis who have this TB problem. Our Mother has saved us from that. She is our protector,' Sushila says.

Sushila wants to talk about issues other than TB. 'See, in this time of Covid, people are already avoiding us. Temples are closed and hence we can't go there. Devotees offer us something or the other and we survive. We cannot take out jag as people don't allow us into their homes and even on the premises because of Covid. We are daughters of Yellamma and still, people are avoiding us,' she says.

'Covid can spread if precaution is not taken,' I point out.

'Yes, yes. Even TB is contagious...I know,' she says, and suddenly tries to change the topic.

'Would you like to have a cup of tea?' she asks me.

When I politely refuse, she asks me to have a cup of milk. When I demur, since I have already had breakfast, she looks crestfallen.

'At least water? Or do you have a problem with even the water in our house?' she asks.

I agree to have some tea. Sushila asks one of the girls to prepare tea with extra milk.

'Yes. You were asking about TB. But really there is no such thing here. We are all healthy and perfect. Our Mother has protected us,' she reiterates.

When Sushila was a child, her grandmother took her to Saundatti, the temple town of Goddess Yellamma in Karnataka. She was married to the Goddess before she attained puberty. 'My grandmother was a devadasi. My family had promised Yellama that they would dedicate me to the Goddess if their wishes were fulfilled. Accordingly, I was handed over to the Goddess and my family members snapped ties with me,' says Sushila.

There is an uncomfortable silence in the room as she narrates her story with a stoic expression. Other devadasis in the room have similar stories about their lives. All of them were married to the Goddess at the ages of seven or ten, and everyone had similar reasons. If they were born as boys, life would have been different, they say.

People need sons to 'take care' of them in their old age and they promise the Goddess to dedicate a daughter if they have a son. Also, many families make a vow to marry a daughter to a goddess if an ailment of some family member is cured. There are many families that have a tradition of dedicating daughters to gods and goddesses. Once married to a goddess, the majority of devadasis are on their own.

'What options do you think we have to live? Men will not spare us even when we are married to the Goddess,' says Shantabai.

Begging and prostitution are the main options for many while others settle down with a malak (literal meaning: owner. A man who looks after a devadasi and treats her as a wife but without marrying her). 'I had a malak. I have two sons from him but they are not legal heirs to the property. My children and I are nowhere on the record. He used to give me some money. But it was not enough,' Sushila says. She curses her parents, grandmother, and even the Goddess. 'When I get angry, I fight with Yellu Aai (Mother Yellamma). I blame her saying, you black-faced woman, you have destroyed my life. I am not even able to live a simple, dignified life because of you...' she says, slapping herself on the forehead.

'My malak left me after using me for five years,' says Hirabai. When she was a child, Hirabai's mother found a sticky, glue-like substance in her daughter's hair while combing it. Family members and neighbours said it was jat—the matted locks of hair considered a symbol of Yellama's presence. Jats are not cleaned. Instead, vermilion, turmeric, and the milky sap of plants are regularly added to the hair. No comb is used and no water applied. It results in heavy, matted locks that become dirtier with time. 'Jat should not be disturbed because it can incur the wrath of the Goddess,' Hirabai says. All of them share their stories but are unwilling to talk about TB or HIV. They have their own reasons to avoid these subjects.

Sacred Lives

Sushila's companion, Shobha, says that the life of a devadasi is sacred as she is the blessed one. 'But society treats us like prostitutes. We become public property and anyone can come and exploit us (for sex),' she complains. Between June and August 2015, SAKHI—Resource Centre for Women conducted a survey in twenty villages of Bellary district in northern Karnataka. The survey studied families of devadasi women with reference to their socio-economic surroundings and found that the spread of HIV-AIDS and TB is becoming rampant among younger girls. Despite tuberculosis being identified as 'a major disease prevalent among these groups there is no data to ascertain exactly how many people are affected by the disease', the survey reported.[1]

One of the most dangerous threats for devadasis is AIDS. They have multiple sexual partners and yet, there is low awareness about issues related to personal hygiene. Most suffer from reproductive tract infections and sexually transmitted diseases. In Mumbai (the capital of Maharashtra), these women were found with several forms of venereal disease and an estimated 20% of the devadasis are infected with HIV, according to the report, titled 'Exploitation of Women as Devadasis and its Associated Evils'. The two-volume report, submitted to the National Commission for Women (NCW), New Delhi, has been authored by Dr V. Bharathi Harishankar and Dr M. Priyamvadha. The report mentions a survey in Karnataka, which found that 26% of female sex workers enter the profession through the devadasi system.

Most devadasis struggle to develop healthy sexual practices, and have to grapple with the stigma of their profession, HIV, and other Sexually Transmitted Diseases (STDs).[2]

Sadhana Zadbuke, a veteran activist who has worked with devadasis for over two decades, says that she has come across many cases where devadasis were infected with HIV and TB. 'Devadasis are still away from the health system. Their overall living conditions are not good, especially devadasis in rural areas live in abject poverty. They are exploited at each and every step of life. They are called women of the Goddess, but they are victims of social tradition.' She adds that the majority of devadasis do not pay attention to their health. There are two reasons. Once they are identified as HIV or TB infected, they are stigmatised. And they fear losing their occupation. Devadasis also fear that their malaks will desert them and those working as commercial sex workers fear they will lose customers from the stigma of HIV or TB. Activists are worried that many of the devadasis try to conceal TB and HIV and continue to work without availing any treatment.

Says an activist working with these women, 'One of the devadasis was working in my home as a maid. Once, she was not well and I asked her to go for a check-up. It was TB. She left the job fearing that I might force her to avail treatment.'

'Surviving is the only aim of our lives. Almost all devadasis are from backward castes. You will not find any devadasi who is from the upper caste. The government gives us Rs 1,000 pension per month but it is not regular. Many malaks abandon devadasis whenever they want and we have to look for other support. Our children have no fathers,' says Champa, a devadasi, explaining why they avoid treatment in government hospitals. 'Health is the last thing on our minds. Life is a mess and who wants to live? What is the value of our so-called sacred life?' she asks.

As Sushila and her companions continue to insist that whatever has happened to their lives is Yellamma's wish, Javed, a young eunuch, enters the room.

'This Goddess follows you wherever you go. She doesn't recognise you as a Hindu or a Muslim. She drags you towards her. I have experienced it,' says Javed. He claims that he was sexually abused by his close relatives when he was a child. 'I knew that I was different. And in school, children tortured me. I became more and more aggressive as I grew up,' he says.

While speaking to me, Javed reveals the 'rate' for sex with a eunuch. 'What should we do to live?' he asks. Sushila intervenes and says that Javed is not jogta (eunuch dedicated to Yellama) but has been with the devadasis helping them to resolve their problems.

Javed is vocal. 'Yes. It is a fact that devadasis and eunuchs face a lot of health issues and we don't get enough treatment and support. There is a need for proper counselling and outreach. But the first thing is that society must acknowledge our presence and admit us as its members. We are disposable, like "use-and-throw". If you don't treat us as equals, as human beings, why should we bother about you and why should you bother about our health?' He says that the community in Sangli and Kolhapur districts must get better health facilities along with assistance, but this will not happen until government bureaucrats are sensitised on how to treat devadasis and eunuchs. Sangli and Kolhapur districts have a number of devadasis working as commercial sex workers. Sangli was once known as an HIV hotspot due to the high number of HIV infections in its redlight areas. The district is on the border of Karnataka and many devadasis from Saundatti, in the neighbouring State, land up, becoming prostitutes here.

In Search of Light

The government health machinery, law, police, and society have exploited the devadasi community. In fact, in drought-prone areas of Maharashtra and Karnataka, the tradition of dedicating girls to the Goddess continues unabated despite various laws being passed by States to ban it.

But there are individuals like Sitavva who are trying hard to end this tradition. Sitavva Joddati gained name and fame in 2018 when the Central government awarded her the Padma Shri, a coveted civilian award. At the age of seven, Sitavva was dedicated as a devadasi by her parents as they wanted to have a son with the blessings of the Goddess. As Sitavva was trying to analyse the system of exploitation, she realised that she needed to do something to save the lives of girls. Since 1991, she has been working with activists and people active in social movements. She garnered the support of other devadasis and joined the Mahila Abhivrudhi Samrakshana Sansthe (MASS), an organization working for devadasis. Over the years, Sitavva has rescued thousands of women and girls from the devadasi practice and helped them gain skills to earn a livelihood. Whenever they receive information about a devadasi dedication, her group members reach the spot to prevent it and save the girls.

Sushila and other devadasis in her group are aware of the exploitative system and the efforts to eradicate it. But they struggle to come to terms with the bitter truths of life. Why does a Goddess like girls from backward communities? If devadasis are close to the Goddess, why do men exploit them? As women of the Goddess, why do they have no respect in society? Why do hundreds of devadasis die of AIDS, TB, and other diseases without treatment? There are many questions that need to be raised, discussed, and debated.

Sushila bows her head and grows silent. There are many who have stories to share, but ultimately decide not to speak as the stories are the same even if their names are different. One of the women in the group, who looks feeble, has tears in her eyes. She remains silent throughout the conversation, trying to control her cough. As tears flow, she starts gasping for breath. She wants to speak but cannot because of her cough. 'Don't worry, we are with you,' Sushila assures her.

After a lull, Sushila starts singing the praises of Yellamma. The others join in unconsciously. They continue to sing with expressionless faces, almost as if they know that their Mother may not have solutions to many of their problems. They will have to find those answers themselves.

NOTES

1. SAKHI-Resource Centre for Women. Retrieved from https://www.globalgiving.org/pfil/33734/projdoc.pdf
2. Harishankar, V & Priyamvadha, M. (2016). Exploitation of Women as Devadasis and its Associated Evils. Retrieved from http://ncwapps.nic.in/pdfReports/Exploitation_of_Women_as_Devadasis_and_its_Associated_Evils_Report.pdf

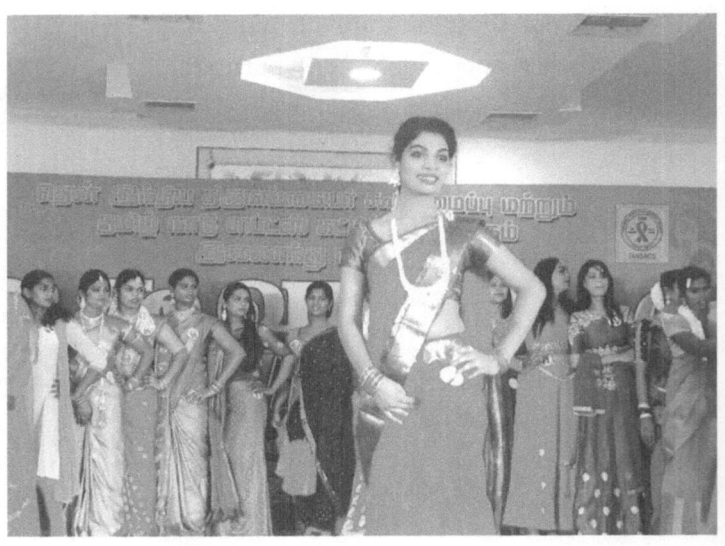

Transgenders participating in the Miss Koovagam competition at Villupuram organized by the Tamil Nadu State AIDS Control Society. The contest has helped to break the stereotypical image of transgenders. General knowledge, social awareness, and the contestants' contribution to the future of the community are also part of the requirements of the event.
(picture credit: Tamil Nadu State AIDS Control Society)

7

Transgenders and TB: Trapped Souls

As the sun goes down on the horizon and dusk sets in, Soumya tries to find her way to the temple premises along a dusty road. There is a big crowd around her and Soumya, draped in a red sari and wearing a sleeveless blouse, artificial gold bangles, and a glittering necklace, is unable to find her friends. She gasps as she makes her way through the crowd. Uncomfortable as sweat rolls down her brow ruining her heavy make-up, Soumya pushes back at the surging crowd and shouts at those who are deliberately trying to jostle her. 'Come and take off my sari and take me right here, you scoundrels. Have you not seen a beautiful woman? Don't you have a mother and sister at home?' she screams in Tamil at a middle-aged man. He grins at her with lustful eyes before disappearing into the crowd. Soumya continues to rage at him.

By the time she reaches the temple premises, many men have been at the receiving end of her fury. She finally finds her friends waiting for her near the temple and sits down by a tree near a flower stall, exhausted from the ordeal. She leans against the tree and drinks some water as her friends rally around her.

Soumya and her friends along with hundreds of others will get married in a short while in a mass ceremony on this full moon day. There is a huge crowd around the temple.

There are dozens of small sacred fires burning within the temple premises. A little later, Soumya and her friends are married, and proudly wear mangalsutras, the marker of a married woman, around their necks. The ceremony is completed in just a few minutes. They have all married the same groom, Aravan, who is not with them but inside the temple. Soumya and the others start dancing and clapping their hands after the marriage ceremony. They hug each other in congratulations. 'Now, my friends will have their honeymoon,' Soumya declares. 'Hope you don't want to join the honeymoon. If not, let's talk. I am free now to answer all your questions, Mr Reporter,' she says with a disarming smile.

Her friends, meanwhile, are talking to men keen to

have sex without protection. There is some bargaining for a few minutes and then they depart with their partners for the nearby fields. Soumya cuts a path through the crowd and moves towards a small tin-shed shop a good distance away from the temple.

'Oh! I forgot to introduce you to my husband. Have you seen him? He looks gorgeous with his huge mustache. You can see him tomorrow. He will come out of the temple,' Soumya says excitedly. As we walk among the crowd, it is late night, and the entire area has turned into an open ground for sex.

The Village of Koothandavar

Welcome to Koovagam, a dusty village in Kallakurichi district, Tamil Nadu, about 200 kms south of Chennai, the State's capital. The village comes alive every year in the month of Chitirai (April/May) with thousands of transgender community members arriving there to marry Lord Aravan (Koothandavar). The festival is significant for transgenders or Aravanis (as they are known in Tamil Nadu), for various religious, cultural, and social reasons. This is the day transgenders identify themselves with the reincarnation of Lord Krishna. Legend has it that in the Mahabharata, a young warrior called Aravan, Arjuna's son, was to be sacrificed at the altar of war so that the Pandavas could defeat the Kauravas. A day before he was to be sacrificed, Aravan expressed a desire to marry, but no girl was willing to become a widow a day after marriage. It was then that Lord Krishna took the form of Mohini and married Aravan. And so, the transgender community in Tamil Nadu and in many parts of India identify themselves with the Mohini avatar of Krishna. They marry Aravan on a full-moon day and become widows the next day, as Aravan dies.

'This is the day we experience a sense of dignity as we feel like we are a reincarnation of the God,' says Soumya. She gasps as she enters the rear of the paan and flower shop. The shopkeeper knows her. 'Come, you people can sit here and talk. I shall send you a cup of tea,' he offers, leading the way to a room inside.

'Please sit at a distance,' she requests. 'Otherwise, you will print a story that Soumya, a transgender, infected a reporter with HIV and TB. And that, too, without having sex. Anyway, you people are more interested in preaching to us about HIV and TB than understanding the reality of our lives,' she laughs.

'Do you have HIV and TB?' I ask.

'Ha! Ha! I have everything in my life. It's a perfect movie with all the masala, emotions, and fights. But who is interested in my life? I must thank you for showing interest in speaking to me. Otherwise, I am a sex doll and especially today, nobody is interested in talking. Everybody just wants to have sex. We are sex-hungry people,' she says, speaking without pausing to catch her breath.

Soumya shies away from sharing details about her family and her background but reveals that she realised she was 'different' while in school. Soumya found she had 'girlish feelings'. In the eighth standard, she told her mother that she wanted to wear a girl's dress, prompting her mother to beat her. She was taken to a spiritual guru, who told her parents that their boy had been cursed by God and some rituals had to be performed to appease Him. But nothing changed after the rituals. One day, she ran away from home to become Soumya. She became a beggar, living on the streets of Chennai. A group of transgenders spotted Soumya on the streets and introduced her to a new world.

'It was the beginning of a new life. It has been over fifteen years now and I am living my own life,' she declares. Commercial sex work has been her main occupation over the years. 'I wanted to find a job. But nobody gave me one. I was ready to work as a domestic help or a sweeper. Anything...But people ridiculed me. Nobody gives jobs to transgenders. How should we survive?' She is visibly disturbed. 'Transgenders have a soul, a heart, and emotions, and are not just a body that can be used whenever people want to satisfy their lust,' Soumya says in a voice choked with emotion. She has fought hard with her family, society, and her own self to counter prejudices and establish her identity as a woman.

'You have come to study HIV because the government and NGOs are focusing on it. But HIV and TB are not new to us. They have become part of our lives. We have accepted it and have to live with it,' she says.

The incidence of TB in transgender persons is not known and needs to be measured. The Revised National TB Control Programme (RNTCP) records the gender of service seekers under three categories: women, men, and transgenders. In 2018, a total of 1,676 transgender persons were diagnosed with TB and this was notified in the RNTCP.[1]

HIV and TB, the Siblings

A few years ago, Soumya was detected with HIV. She says that she did not receive proper treatment, and after developing a persistent cough and fever, was diagnosed with pulmonary TB.

'I am finding it difficult to survive. No prostitution for me now because of these ailments. I have saved some money but I don't want to spend all of it on my treatment. The government says there is free treatment, but it is all bakwaas (nonsense). We don't get timely treatment and medicines,' she complains.

Soumya says that God—her husband Aravan—gave her HIV. It is not surprising that Soumya contracted TB immediately after contracting HIV. 'A doctor told me that if you have HIV, you will get TB. HIV and TB are like siblings. They can't live without each other,' she says.

Overcome with emotion, she suddenly bursts into tears. 'Don't know why, but today I am remembering my sister and my parents. I have no idea how they are...' Unable to speak, she pauses for a few moments. '...But I feel that I have every right to live my own life,' she resumes. 'I felt like a girl's soul was trapped in a boy's body and my parents and society were not ready to accept me in this form. I feel one should not allow anyone, not even parents, to control one's life. And that's why I left my home. Freedom comes at a price and I have paid a heavy price.'

Soumya says that she can sense death approaching and that TB has accelerated her journey towards the end.

According to the World Health Organization (WHO), people living with HIV are eighteen times more likely to develop active TB than people without HIV. This is a lethal combination, with each speeding the other's progress. In 2019, about 2,08,000 people died of HIV-associated TB across the world. In 2019, 69% of notified TB patients had a documented HIV test result, up from 64% in 2018.[2]

God's Widow

Late at night, Soumya's just-married friends return with a rich haul. They say they have had 'several honeymoons', and Soumya bursts into laughter. The next morning, Soumya and her friends are gearing up for the widowhood ceremony. The lavish make-up, wigs, dresses, and staccato clapping are all gone. There is wailing all around. All the transgenders queue up in front of a man wearing a garland. The man holds a knife and cuts a yellow thread that the transgenders had worn around their necks the previous day, during the marriage ceremony. After cutting the thread, he breaks the bangles on their hands. Some pretend to cry, some genuinely wail in distress.

'This is the last one. No marriage and no widowhood for me next year,' says Soumya.

'Why?' I ask.

'Enough of this. Such things are not going to lead me anywhere in life. My ailments have taught me a lesson and I want to save my sisters from what I have gone through. There is no proper treatment for the poor. The government hospitals treat us like trash. There is less of treatment and more of insults. You know what, once, a compounder at a government hospital asked why I was taking HIV treatment and what is the use of life for people like us. He said that the government should spend money on treating normal people.'

'What was your reply? You should have registered a complaint,' I say.

'Let it be, reporter-ji. No need. I didn't give him any reply. But I shall tell you what my answer is.' As we walked away from the temple, Soumya told me about her plans. She was trying to connect with NGOs so that transgenders could acquire professional skills that can help them get jobs. She wants to use the money she has saved on her friends so that they can complete their education in an open university. 'This is my reply to society's obnoxious treatment of my community. I am going to fight for our rights,' she insists.

The Government of India's National Framework for a Gender-Sensitive Responsive Approach to TB in India states that social distance from the health system, poor access to health care, and stigma are concerns among transgenders.

The stigma for transgenders is threefold: social discrimination as a transgender; discrimination because of being a transgender with TB; discrimination for being a transgender person with HIV and TB or presumed to have HIV. 'Transgender persons often have low literacy, low education levels, and are poor. A high proportion of transgender persons are known to smoke, consume alcohol, and use drugs.

All these factors make them vulnerable to TB,' the National Framework document adds, mentioning that poor health literacy and fear of criminalisation create hurdles for transgender persons to seek treatment. Undernutrition and poor health literacy adds to the risk of TB and diagnosis is delayed because of poor access to healthcare and a perceived lack of privacy in the health system. Overcrowded houses with poor ventilation lead to higher and sustained exposure to the infection, the report adds.[3]

Dignity is Development

Soumya admits that she consumes alcohol and sometimes uses drugs. 'But don't focus on this. Write something about how people treat us. We are human beings. We beg and become prostitutes because you people force us to do so. Society wants us to live this way. Just as we need treatment for TB and HIV, your society needs mental treatment so it understands how to treat human beings,' Soumya adds, trying to end the conversation.

'Where do I send you the published story? Any address?' I ask her.

She smiles. 'No need. What I will do with your story? I know you will write a true story,' she says, taking a deep breath.

'And what if I want to meet you again?' I enquire.

'No, sir. You can't. We met because you came to Koovagam. And even if you come to Koovagam next time, I will not be here,' she says with finality.

Soumya is determined to live a life with no strings attached to the outer world. She is keen to ensure that her friends live a better life than her.

I press on. 'Can I at least help you connect with NGOs or other groups that will help you to do something for your community?'

'No, thank you. Don't consider me weak. I am a strong person and I will find a way to make life better for my community. I want to earn the status of human beings for all of us,' she says with folded hands.

As we leave, a colleague accompanying me warns me not to become emotional about Soumya and believe her 'drama'.

Entering the world of the transgender community is not easy and hence tracking transgenders with HIV or TB is one of the toughest tasks the health machinery has to face. The community lives in ghettos and has its own rules and regulations.

'It is the guru who decides what I should and should not do. Any decision about my life will be guided by my guru, who gave me entry into the community,' says Janesar. She adds that she is able to survive because of the tightly-knit community. There is no entry for people from the other world, be they doctors or the police. 'The government people who are supposed to help us exploit us,' says Janesar. 'We can only believe in God and rely on him to help us. When our parents don't want us, what can we expect from society and the government?' she asks.

Many, like Janesar, are in Koovagam to participate in a beauty contest, which has become the centre of attraction. This contest, which has helped to smash stereotypes, is exclusively for transgenders and the governmental and other agencies sponsoring events on the occasion focus on health issues.

Before leaving the village, I visited the temple to see Aravan. He looked fierce with his big moustache. But he was still and unaffected by the sufferings inflicted by the world on his wives. Perhaps it was not surprising then, that one of his wives had decided to leave him forever and live on her own.

NOTES

1. Central TB Division, Ministry of Health and Family Welfare. (2019). National Framework for a Gender—Responsive approach to TB in India. Retrieved from—https://tbcindia.gov.in/WriteReadData/l892s/388838054811%20NTEP%20Gender%20Responsive%20Framework_311219.pdf
2. World Health Organization. (2020). Tuberculosis. Retrieved from—https://www.who.int/news-room/fact-sheets/detail/tuberculosis
3. Central TB Division, Ministry of Health and Family Welfare. (2019). National Framework for a Gender—Responsive approach to TB in India. Retrieved from—https://tbcindia.gov.in/WriteReadData/l892s/388838054811%20NTEP%20Gender%20Responsive%20Framework_311219.pdf

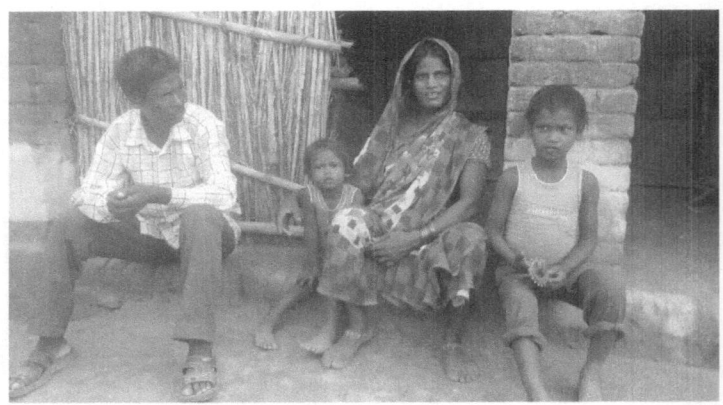

Arjun, with his father Phulwari Prasad and mother Usha, in Semara Hardo village, Uttar Pradesh. The struggle for survival is a daily battle for Musahars. *(picture credit: Radheshyam Jadhav)*

8

Nutrition and TB: Living on Rats

Little Arjun has a battle on his hands. Nothing distracts the child, whose facial expressions are like that of a warrior at Kurukshetra. He runs around with a small sack and a lathi (stick) in his hands. His mother Usha and father Phulwari Prasad are sitting on the threshold of their hut, proudly watching their warrior.

'Our kid is grown up now. He is worried about us and I am sure he will feed us tonight,' says Usha, trying to smile. She calls out to Arjun saying that guests have come to meet the family. 'Now, come here and sit with us. This sahib will click our picture.'

Arjun unwillingly drops the lathi and sack to clutch his mother's hand while sitting beside her. There is complete silence for a few moments as Usha and Phulwari are unwilling to speak. Eventually, Usha says, 'He (Arjun) was catching rats for our dinner. What to do? You people find it strange, but for us it is normal.' Arjun is embarrassed. He hangs his head and casts a glance at his mother.

People from Semara Hardo village in Uttar Pradesh's Kushinagar district often come to Musahar Toli, outside their village, to watch what they call the 'circus of rat catching and eating'. Arjun does not like people laughing at him. Usha holds him closer and tells the boy that the guests are here to speak to the family and not to watch how they catch and eat rats. But Arjun refuses to look up.

'Arey, why are you afraid? Tell me how you eat roasted rats. Say something. Tell us how rats taste,' says a young political aspirant from the village, who is accompanying me. Now, Phulwari chips in to save his family from further embarrassment.

'Sahib, we are poor, helpless people. We hardly get any work. We don't have a regular income and hence our food habits are different. Why would we eat rats? You tell us,' he says with folded hands. 'It is not that we eat rats daily. But sometimes, when we don't have anything to eat...' Arjun is impatient now. He is not interested in talking. From the corner of his eye, he looks at a dark room. He has probably spied a rat and is waiting for us to go away.

Usha contradicts her husband. She says that rats

and ghonga (snails) are part of their regular diet. But this is not an exception. Almost every family in the basti (slum) eats rats and snails.

People in the basti say that many of the Musahars of Musahar Toli have succumbed to starvation and ailments for years. However, the destitution and hunger of the Musahars, who live in primitive conditions, attracts little or no attention. Musahars are called Mahadalits, because their socio-economic life is worse than that of Dalits. 'Musahar', the community's name, is a distortion of mushak ahari (rat eater). The community is concentrated in Bihar, Jharkhand, Madhya Pradesh, and Uttar Pradesh.

For years, Musahar localities have suffered Visceral Leishmaniasis (VL), a vector-borne parasitic disease, Japanese encephalitis and TB. Starvation is common in their squalid localities, which are ghettos on village borders with people living in unhealthy conditions. Many succumb without a diagnosis of their ailments and without treatment. Deaths due to starvation and TB are common but nothing is on the record, allege activists.

'When there are frequent deaths, sometimes government babus come for a check-up. They take us to the government hospital and give us some tablets. That's all. But it is a fact that we struggle to earn enough to feed our families. Some work in brick kilns, some have hand carts, and many work as labourers. Life here is all about the struggle to earn two meals a day,' says Phulwari.

A WHO document entitled 'Addressing Poverty in TB Control: Options for National TB Control Programmes' states that TB symptoms may be neglected in the poor as they start gradually and the poor regularly suffer from intercurrent diseases. Work is vital for survival and health is not a priority. 'This, coupled with a lack of knowledge about TB, may lead patients to dismiss symptoms as unimportant or to attribute them to other conditions such as a chronic cough or prolonged influenza,' the WHO report states.

Illiteracy and low levels of education lead to further lack of awareness about the importance of early diagnosis and treatment of TB. The poor may be unaware of TB treatment, which is widely available and often free of charge, the WHO states, adding that deprived communities might have different degrees of knowledge about and attitudes towards TB. The poor in urban slum areas and in remote rural areas may view TB in different ways, it states.[1]

As the discussions between the adults go on, Arjun loses his patience. He gets up and picks up a stick to kill a rat. Arjun does not go to school. His classmates tease him about being a rat eater. Like Arjun, there are many children in the locality. Not surprisingly, Usha and Phulwari have not stopped their son from catching rats. From their point of view, he will have at least one way to get food. He should not die of starvation, asserts Usha.

'Pappu and Feku Died of TB'

'There is no starvation. People have died of TB and TB has nothing to do with starvation. You people are unnecessarily creating a ruckus,' a village elder from the upper-caste community says, as we enter the Musahar basti of Jungle Khirkia village. He says that the government gives many 'free' things to the poor, including foodgrain, and there is no reason for them to die of starvation. The old man makes every effort to convince us that the deaths in Musahar basti are because of TB.

Government posters with information about TB are pasted all over the basti walls. The village came into the limelight in 2018 after two Musahar siblings, Pappu (16) and Feku (22), who were bedridden for months, succumbed one after the other. Government officials said the duo had died of TB, but their mother, Sonwa Devi, claimed that they had died of starvation. With the deaths of her children turned into a political controversy, there has been a steady stream of political leaders visiting the basti to meet Sonwa Devi.

'Now, I am not even able to cry. My tears have

dried up. My sons had turned into skeletons and were completely bedridden. Feku was not able to get out of bed for six months and then, Pappu was also bedridden. They worked in a brick kiln but were not able to go to work for months because they were weak. We had food sometimes and many a time, we went to sleep on empty stomachs,' says Sonwa Devi, sitting in the courtyard of her brick house.

She says that the doctors had not been able to diagnose what had happened to her sons. 'People in the government hospital asked for money to admit my sons. Feku was admitted after I pleaded, but he died within a few hours. Pappu died the same night. They died without food and treatment.' The government hospital doctors told her that her sons had TB and it was in the last stage.

'I don't know. I only know that I have lost my sons,' she says, looking towards the sky and rapping herself on the head with both hands. Her husband had died about twenty years earlier, leaving behind four sons. Her other two sons, Sanju and Bigu, work as daily-wage labourers. They are married and live separately. 'I have not had any work under the government scheme (Mahatma Gandhi National Rural Employment Guarantee Scheme, MGNREGS). I earn Rs 60 a day whenever I get work. But work is available for hardly 10-12 days a month. You tell me, what do we eat and how are we to live?' she asks.

Uttar Pradesh Chief Minister Yogi Adityanath declared that the two brothers had not died of hunger. They had ration cards and their death was due to TB, he asserted. The chief minister added that a probe was underway to find out whether they had received free TB treatment available under the Directly Observed Treatment Short-course (DOTS) strategy for TB patients. Adityanath said his government had provided housing, ration cards, and job cards to members of the Musahar community, and that the administration was investigating the cause of the deaths. The government is working to ensure that the benefits of welfare schemes reach even the very last person in society, the chief minister claimed, after the deaths of Pappu and Feku came to light in 2018.[2]

Kushinagar's chief medical officer reported that Sonwa Devi's sons had died of cardiorespiratory failure and had pulmonary tuberculosis, while one also had poliomyelitis. But the TB officer from Padrauna block said that tests done by him revealed no such thing. Deaths due to TB were politically safer than deaths caused by starvation, and the State government was keen to prove that TB prevails in Musahar bastis.

But for hundreds of Musahars, death from starvation and TB go hand in hand.

According to the WHO, undernutrition is an important risk factor for TB and TB causes undernutrition. This bi-directional association results in the high prevalence of undernutrition among TB patients. Normal weight and nutrition can be restored with the help of proper TB treatment. 'However, the time to full nutritional recovery can be long and many TB patients are still undernourished after TB treatment is completed. Therefore, it is important to do a nutritional assessment at the time of TB diagnosis and provide nutritional care accordingly,' the WHO states. Proper nutrition is important for the undernourished to reduce general health risks. Food insecurity is a barrier in accessing and adhering to TB treatment as the catastrophic costs of TB and its care can increase food insecurity. The vicious circle of underlying vulnerability leading to TB, and TB leading to aggravated vulnerability, continues.

There is no conclusive evidence that food support is an enabler in accessing and adhering to TB treatment. 'However, experiences suggest that food support can be a critical component of enablers and social protection packages, especially in food-insecure populations,' according to the WHO.[3]

Where is Food for the Poor Going?

Food security, nutrition, vitamins, and protein are words that are alien to Musahars. In Rakba Dulma Patti village, Virendra Musahar and his family find some solace even in the midst of grief. 'We have food to eat,' says ten-year-old Laxmi, while feeding her brother Sunnu (2), who gulps down rice mixed with dal and nags his sister to feed him quickly instead of wasting time talking. Four-year-old Sita waits for her turn as her father Virendra uncovers foodgrain stacked in his one-room house in the stinking, filthy lane. Virendra's wife Sangeeta (30) and their six-year-old son Shyam died on the same day, while his two-month-old daughter Geeta died a few days later. The government record cites diarrhoea as the reason for their deaths, but Virendra and his three malnourished children have a different story to tell. He admits that the family survives on 'anything that can be eaten'.

While coughing, Virendra says that he had to sell his pushcart a few months ago as the family was struggling to survive. A few years ago, Virendra's other son, Laxman, had died with similar symptoms. He was just ten. Virendra started working as a daily-wage labourer but found work only for a few days. His wife Sangeeta had registered herself as an MGNREGS worker, but her card is empty as she did not get any work. Virendra shows a tattered ration card saying that he gets rations, but they are insufficient. But the deaths in the family have fetched some money and foodgrain.

'The district magistrate has given 10,000 rupees;

the sub-divisional officer, 5,000; and the supply officer, 1,000. Also, they have given us a lot of foodgrain,' says Virendra, adding that his wife and son had started vomiting after eating rancid rice. 'Government doctors made me run here and there without treating my wife and son. Doctors at the block hospital asked me to take her to the district hospital even when I could see that she was dead,' he says. Virendra himself coughs and gasps regularly, but has not visited the hospital. He is more worried about what will happen to his kids once the foodgrain provided by the government runs out. He and many others complain that they have not been getting their quota of foodgrain under the public distribution system.

An internal audit by the food and logistics department detected pilferage of 2.2 lakh tonnes of wheat via 1.86 lakh fraudulent transactions in 43 districts of Uttar Pradesh in 2018. The case was given to a special task force because of the technicalities involved and the breadth of the scam. 'Many of us can't read and write. We believe that the shop owner gives our quota of ration every month,' says Mamata, a Musahar woman from Jungle Khirkia village. Prabhawati, another woman from the same village, says that the shop owner claims that every month he gives them 35 kgs under the Antyodaya Anna Yojana. 'We are seven members in the family and the foodgrain suffices only for 10-15 days,' she says. Under the National Food Security Act, 2013 (NFSA), eligible households, which comprise households covered under the Antyodaya Anna Yojana and priority households, are entitled to receive foodgrain (rice, wheat or coarse grains or any combination thereof) at highly subsidised prices. But the ration that the poor are supposed to get finds its way to cities, to be sold in the market. Often, poor Musahars sell their quota to city people as they need money for their other requirements.

Ramrati Devi's Answer

Octogenarian Ramrati Devi, a resident of Malwabar Musahar basti who is no more, saw many starvation/TB deaths in her community. She believed she had a solution. 'We must protect our land. The land is not to sell but to cultivate,' the wise woman insisted. For nearly a decade, this illiterate woman fought against the moneylender who wanted to snatch away her land in lieu of a loan he had given her. Ramrati fought her battle at the community level, with her family, and finally won in court.

She walked 35-40 kms to the district headquarters, Deoria, to meet her lawyer. Ramrati's logic was simple. She believed that land was the only resource that could save her community from starvation and malnutrition. She had no faith in the government's public distribution system but was confident that the community could grow its own food and take the surplus to the market.

'Ramrati Devi knew that the land would not only bring food, but also give them dignity to live life as human beings. She was harassed in every possible way to give up her land. But she refused to succumb. Not many Musahars have land and those who do are pressurised to sell it to the village's upper-caste landlords,' says activist Vidya Bhushan Rawat, who works with the Musahar community in Malwabar. 'The fight is against poverty. The fight against malnutrition and TB is difficult. One has to find a sustainable answer to poverty,' he adds. Rawat has started a centre called Prerna Kendra in Malwabar along with members of the Musahar community.

Ramrati died in December 2020 but her fight has inspired other Musahars, who are keen to protect their land.

*

It is late evening in Malwabar and Sangeeta Kushwaha is working in Prerna Kendra, nudging a couple of Musahar girls to fetch their books and start studying. They speak in a local dialect and Sangeeta translates. 'I want to study and get a job in a city. I know that I have to study if I have to become something,' says the little girl. But it is not going to be easy for her as education remains the lowest priority for the community. A picture of 19th-century social revolutionary Savitribai Phule hangs on the walls of Prerna Kendra. Inspired by her, these Musahar girls are gearing up to lock horns with their oppressors. But it will be a long battle, by far longer and more difficult than the one Arjun is fighting in Semara Hardo.

NOTES

1. World Health Organization (2005). Addressing Poverty in TB Control. Retrieved from https://www.who.int/tb/publications/tb-control-poverty/en/
2. Bano, A. (2018). Musahar brothers did not die of hunger, says CM Yogi. Retrieved from https://timesofindia.indiatimes.com/city/lucknow/musahar-brothers-did-not-die-of-hunger-says-cm-yogi/articleshow/65853223.cms
3. World Health Organization. (2013). Nutritional Care and Support for Patients with Tuberculosis. Retrieved from https://www.who.int/tb/nutrition/en/

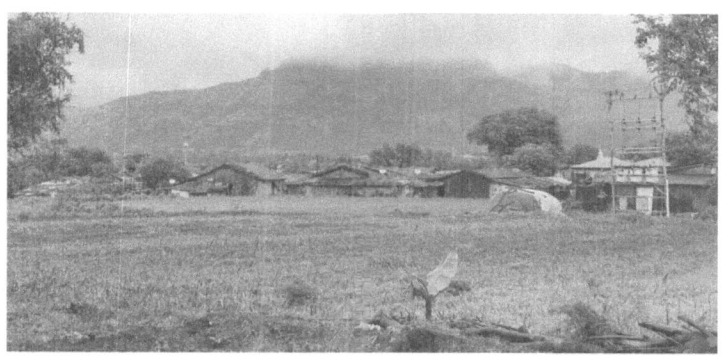

Hausabai's village in a remote part of Nashik district, Maharashtra is silent about her TB and her death.
(picture credit: Radheshyam Jadhav)

9

Tribals and TB: The Trail

The newly renovated Primary Health Centre (PHC) in one of the tribal villages in north Maharashtra is crowded with tribal community members lining up for the Covid-19 vaccine jab. Many of them have questions about the vaccine and the local medical staff try to answer their queries. As the vaccination drive continues in the courtyard, a young TB patient enters the medical officer's room along with an ASHA (accredited social health activist) worker.

The young man, wearing a soiled shirt, tattered trousers, and a red cap, looks pale. He is not comfortable wearing a mask. As he sits silently in a corner, the medical officer and his staff explain how difficult it is for them to track TB patients in remote tribal areas. The Covid-19 outbreak has added to the problems in identifying TB patients. 'We tried to reach village leaders to spread the message that everyone should take the vaccine. Earlier, we had roped in barbers to identify TB patients in the village,' says the officer.

The ASHA worker joins the conversation. 'It is not easy to reach remote localities. Sometimes, we have to walk 15-20 kms as there is no road. He (the young man with TB) was not willing to come to the centre. The last time he came for tests his sputum test was positive.' She is worried about falling short of the TB patient identification target set for her. The ASHA worker gets Rs 500 as an incentive for each new patient she identifies.

The young man is restless as the medical officer asks him if he takes his tablets regularly. After a few minutes, he asks the young man to narrate his story but gets no response. The discussions go on for about an hour, and the young man remains a silent listener throughout. When the discussions are about to end, he finally pipes up to enquire if the government is providing any employment for tribals in the region.

'Farming is the only source of livelihood and it depends on the monsoon. The majority of us migrate to cities to work as construction workers or take whatever work is available. Government work (under the Mahatma Gandhi National Rural Employment

Scheme) is not regularly available. Life has become more difficult due to Covid-19,' he says.

Slowly gaining confidence that he will not be used as a guinea pig, he starts to talk about TB. 'My sister was not feeling well and we took her to the bhagat (local godman). He said that she would be okay after receiving his treatment. He performed a ritual, but even after weeks, my sister was not normal. Her cough and fever grew worse and we decided to approach this hospital. Doctors said she had TB and needed immediate treatment. We started the medicine but also continued to seek the bhagat's guidance.'

Even as his sister was recovering, the young man began to suffer from a sore throat, fever, and weakness. 'I habitually consume liquor made out of the Mahua flower. I increased my liquor consumption and felt better. But then the fever crippled me. ASHA tai (sister) asked me to have a check-up and I was diagnosed with TB. I am taking treatment regularly and the doctor sahib has said I will recover in six months,' he says.

Treatment Tale

After the young man departs, the medical officer expresses doubts about whether he will complete the treatment. 'Awareness about TB is very low and the low standard of living, poor nutrition, and overall backwardness make them vulnerable to many diseases. In these areas, the local bhagat is the first doctor for any patient and we are trying to reach all these bhagats. Every hamlet has one bhagat each,' says the officer.

In one locality, the bhagat told people that TB treatment is not required as he can treat TB with rituals and traditional medicines. 'He was influential and people stopped coming to us. But one day, he himself fell ill and was not able to recover using his methods. He came to the PHC and was diagnosed with TB. We told him that he should not risk his and others' lives,' says the medical assistant at the PHC. The bhagat and his followers were treated at the PHC. But at the same time, the bhagat continued to 'treat' people.

TB is very much a stigma among the tribal people and there are many instances of family members kicking out infected patients, says a senior treatment supervisor, who has been working with the TB programme as a contract employee for the last twenty years. He added that there is a karbhari (headman) in every hamlet who takes the majority of the decisions for the community and the individuals.

The main tribes in Maharashtra are the Bhils, Gonds, Mahadeo Kolis, Pawras, Thakars, Varlis, Kolams, Katkaris, and Madia Gonds. These are close-knit communities concentrated in the hilly parts of Maharashtra, including Dhule, Nandurbar, Jalgaon, Nashik, and Thane. They also have a presence in the eastern forest districts of Chandrapur, Gadchiroli, Bhandara, Gondia, Nagpur, Amravati, and Yavatmal.

In India, Scheduled Tribe communities live in about 15% of the country's total land area, in various ecological and geoclimatic conditions ranging from plains and forests to hills. Tribal groups are at different stages of social, economic, and educational development, according to the Government of India. While some tribal communities are now part of the mainstream way of life, there are 75 tribes known as Particularly Vulnerable Tribal Groups (PVTGs) who were earlier termed Primitive Tribal Groups and are not part of the mainstream style of life. But TB has penetrated all levels of the community.

The female staff at the PHC say that while the majority of spousal desertion cases involve men abandoning their wives because of TB, there are also cases where women leave their husbands after they are diagnosed with the disease.

Hausabai (name changed) was abandoned by her husband. 'She was diagnosed with TB after marriage. Her husband suspected that she had TB even before the marriage. Hausabai delivered a baby girl and her husband left her at her parents' home. Her brother brought her to us and we started her treatment,' says the medical officer.

'How is she now?' I enquire.

'She has completely recovered. But unfortunately, her husband is not willing to take her back. We tried to convince him. But he is not listening to us.'

'Can we meet Hausabai? Where does she live?' I ask.

'I think she lives with her parents a few kilometres from here. Let me find out,' says the officer, directing two members from his staff to make some calls.

The medical officer claims that people have faith in the government health system and that he and his staff have been making every effort to provide quality treatment and follow up on every TB patient.

One of the staff members who had stepped out of the room to get Hausabai's details comes back after a few minutes.

'Did you get Hausabai's location?' the officer asks.

The staff member's response leaves everyone in the room stunned. 'Hausabai died a few months back. Her brother says she died of TB.'

She Wanted to Live

The small pathway leading to Hausabai's house is full of muck and is slippery. Stepping out of the car on to the main road, the medical officer says he will join us later as he has to visit the vaccination centre at the corner of the road. After walking a few kilometres in the rain, we see Hausabai's home. The local ASHA worker, a young woman who knew Hausabai very well, leads the way. Hausabai's brother stands on the threshold of the house and explains what happened to his sister. As the light rain turns into a downpour, he invites everyone into the small, dank, and dark brick house.

Hausabai's mother rummages through a heap of clothes to find something and shows us a tattered photo album of Hausabai's wedding.

'See, this is my girl. She looks beautiful...See the smile on her face. She wanted to live,' says Kanubai (name changed), placing a trembling finger on her daughter's photo. As she turns page after page of the album, she keeps talking about Hausabai.

'Can you do something for her daughter? She is six years old and her father will not look after her. We are looking after her, but how long can we take care of her?' asks the old woman, with tears in her eyes. Hausabai's daughter is sleeping on the floor in a corner of the room.

Hausabai's brother is a farmer. He takes out a bunch of medical reports and X-rays from the cupboard. 'She was repeatedly falling ill and her weight went down to 27 kgs. She was not eating. I took her to a private hospital in the city. The doctors said that her TB was in the last stage and her lungs were completely damaged. The doctors gave her tablets and asked us to come back for another check-up,' he recounts. 'She was not ready to go to the government hospital. She insisted on visiting a private doctor,' he adds.

While the treatment was on, Hausabai's family members took her to the local bhagat, who extracted Rs 5,000 from the family and gave her a box of sweets. He told them that evil spirits had entered her body and that eating the sweets would drive them away.

'Nothing worked and she was completely bedridden,' says her brother. He believes that her TB was not properly treated. 'We tried our best to save her but failed completely,' he sighs.

'Why didn't you approach us?' asks the government hospital staff member who had accompanied me to Hausabai's home.

'Your mobile number was not reachable sir. I tried several times but...'

'You should have brought her to the PHC. There are many others who would have helped to get her admitted. Private doctors have looted you. The government provides everything for free,' says the staff member.

Hausabai's brother is quiet.

'She has gone now. What is the point in discussing this? Can you help her daughter, at least?' asks Kanubai. No one has a response.

Tracking Tribals

When the Government of India launched the Tribal TB Initiative in 2021, about 177 districts were identified as high-priority districts, where the remote location, malnutrition, poor living conditions, and lack of awareness contribute to the vulnerability of the tribal population to the disease. The Tribal TB initiative is a partnership between the Ministry of Health and Family Welfare and the Ministry of Tribal Affairs to improve the cascade of TB care and support services among Tribal Populations.[1]

There are about 10.4 crore tribals in India, accounting for 8.6% of the total population. The community has a higher prevalence (703 per 1,00,000) of TB compared to the national average of 256 per 1,00,000. '10.4% of all TB notified patients are from tribal communities. The National TB programme has prioritized this subgroup of the population through Tribal Action Plans since 2005,' states the Tribal TB Initiative document.

Geographical locations are major barriers in access, availability, and utilisation of TB care services by tribal communities. There are other issues such as the poor state of social determinants, high impact of malnutrition, insufficient community involvement, health system constraints (such as lack of trained human resources), as well as cultural and communication gaps between the care provider and the community. Covid-19 has worsened the situation, the document states.[2]

'It is not just about TB. It is about the way the tribal population is treated. Every government babu tells us that we need to improve our quality of life by joining the mainstream. But what is mainstream? Should we become like you people?' asks Sunil Pawara. He says that in the name of development, land, water, and forests belonging to tribal communities are being taken over by governments and handed over to corporates. Young people like Sunil are suspicious of any government initiative, saying that their experiences in the past have made them cautious. Not surprisingly, the community has started relying more on its local leaders.

Participatory Approach

Kesari Nelu Telami is a demigod for the tribal community in Morkhandi, a remote, Naxal-affected village in Maharashtra's Gadchiroli district. He is known as a pujari (priest) and he treats tribals with traditional methods, using medicinal plants. People have elected him unopposed to the village panchayat and he is the head of the Devada panchayat. After he questioned the efficacy and need for Covid-19 vaccines, villagers stayed away from the vaccination drive.

Community members believe that poor-quality vaccines were dispatched to their district and good-quality vaccines were reserved for rich people in the cities. Some feared that the vaccines would actually infect them with the Covid-19-causing virus, while others believed that their organs would be removed after they were vaccinated. Many men believed that vaccination would make them impotent.

Many villages are located in a 'liberated zone' loosely overseen by Naxalites. Dense forest and hilly terrain make these villages difficult to access. The Madia tribe here is recognised as a particularly vulnerable tribal group by the Indian government. During the Covid-19 vaccination drive, government officials managed to reach the community, but before any discussion on vaccination, the tribal members drew their attention to basic problems such as lack of water supply. The government officers then approached influential community leaders such as Kesari Nelu Telami and others and tried to bring them on board with the vaccination drive.

Eventually, Telami agreed. While traditional medicinal methods are important, everyone should also take the vaccine, he told community members. He was the first person in the village to get the vaccine and thereafter the entire village lined up for it.[3]

'The top-down approach has failed completely when it comes to spreading awareness about TB or

Covid-19. The government machinery still believes that it can impose things on Adivasis. Any effort should be participatory and people must be convinced. It is a slow process but the only way to reach the community,' says Sunil.

Deciding on Development

Sunil is from the remote Akrani taluka in Nandurbar district, where the majority of villages are completely cut off from other parts of the State. Some of the villagers here had not even set eyes on the Rs 500 and Rs 1,000 notes scrapped by Prime Minister Narendra Modi when he announced the demonetisation drive in 2016. The villagers live in their own world and have their own ways of treating diseases. The current reporting status of smear positive tests suggests that only 11% of pulmonary TB cases in the tribal population get treated.

The report of the expert committee on tribal health in India highlights that adivasis face a triple disease burden. Malnutrition, malaria, and TB are rampant in the community. There has been a rise in the prevalence of non-communicable diseases such as cancer, hypertension, and diabetes because of rapid urbanization, environmental distress, and changing lifestyles. Mental illness, especially addiction, is also rising. The report notes that tribal children continue to be the most malnourished in the country. The prevalence of underweight children is almost one-and-a-half times that of children from other castes.[4]

'The number of malnourished children contracting TB is huge. We are handling more than 100 such cases every year,' says a doctor at one of the PHCs in Nashik. He adds that malnourishment in tribal areas is rising along with poverty.

The erstwhile Planning Commission provided estimates based on Tendulkar Methodology for poverty ratios for the years for which large Sample Surveys on Household Consumer Expenditure have been conducted by the National Sample Survey Office (NSSO) of the Ministry of Statistics and Programme Implementation. 'As per these estimates, Scheduled Tribes (ST) people living below the poverty line in 2011-12 were 45.3% in rural areas and 24.1% in urban areas as compared to 25.7% persons in rural areas and 13.7% persons in urban areas below poverty line for all populations,' states the Government of India's Ministry of Tribal Affairs in its Annual Report 2020-21.

As per the figures published by the Ministry of Health and Family Welfare, there are 28,682 Sub Centres (SCs), 4,211 Primary Health Centres (PHCs), and 1,022 Community Health Centres (CHCs) in tribal areas of India as on 31st March, 2019. At the all-India level there is a shortfall of 7,054 SCs, 1,204 PHCs, and 326 CHCs in tribal areas as compared to the requirement.[5]

In Ahmednagar district's remote Kombhalne village, Rahibai Popere is trying to find a solution to malnourishment so that tribals do not have to rely on hospitals. She has taken a proactive role in the Kalsubai Parisar Biyanee Savardhan Samiti, Akole, an association that is helping farmers to conserve traditional seeds.

Twenty years ago, when her grandson fell ill, Rahibai was convinced vegetables and foodgrains containing 'poison' had made the child unhealthy. She asked her son to stop buying vegetables and foodgrain grown using hybrid seeds, chemicals, and fertilisers. Instead, Rahibai, who has never been to school, started growing local varieties that need just air and water for cultivation.

She established a seed bank in her small mud house for conservation and revival of crop diversity and wild food resources. Rahibai has conserved and multiplied about 43 landraces of seventeen crops (paddy, hyacinth bean, millets, pulses, oilseeds, etc.) by establishing a germplasm conservation centre. She coins her own terms for her agricultural innovations and puts her theories into practice in the field. Rahibai believes that the community has to be clear about what kind of development it requires and then opt for a convergence of modern science and traditional knowledge. The government has acknowledged her work by conferring the Padma Shri civilian Award on her.[6]

NOTES

1. Ministry of Health and Family Welfare. (2021). Dr Harsh Vardhan launches Tribal TB Initiative in pursuit of 'TB Mukt Bharat'. Retrieved from https://pib.gov.in/PressReleasePage.aspx?PRID=1707909
2. Ministry of Health and Family Welfare and Ministry of Tribal Affairs. (2021). Tribal TB Initiative. Retrieved from https://tbcindia.gov.in/WriteReadData/1892s/5883826004Tribal%20TB%20Initiative.pdf
3. Jadhav, R. (2021). Breaking down vaccine hesitancy in Maharashtra's Naxal-affected villages. Retrieved from https://www.thehindubusinessline.com/news/breaking-down-vaccine-hesitancy-in-maharashtras-naxal-affected-villages/article34746562.ece
4. Ministry of Health and Family Welfare and Ministry of Tribal Affairs. (2018). Tribal Health in India. Retrieved from http://nhm.gov.in/nhm_components/tribal_report/Executive_Summary.pdf
5. Ministry of Tribal Affairs. (2020). Annual Report—2020-21. Retrieved from https://tribal.nic.in/downloads/Statistics/AnnualReport/AREnglish2021.pdf
6. Jadhav, R. (2019). 'Seed Mother' who never went to school has lessons for scientists. Retrieved from https://www.thehindubusinessline.com/news/seed-mother-who-never-went-to-school-has-lessons-for-scientists/article26432389.ece

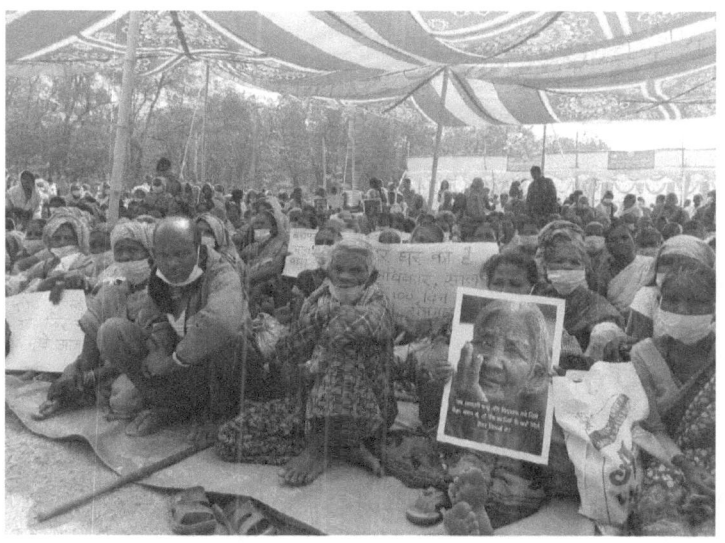

The elderly, single women, and differently abled in Chaibasa (West Singhbhum, Jharkhand). As young people migrate to cities, all of them are left to fight their own battles by themselves. *(representative image. picture credit: Siraj Dutta)*

10

Migration and TB: The Unending Quest

Covid-19-induced lockdowns in 2020 resulted in a massive reverse migration of workers in India. As distressed migrants in cities returned to villages, unemployment rose in an economy that was already stressed. Government data shows that 1.23 crore migrant workers returned to their home states during the Covid-19 lockdown. The actual number, however, could be much higher. This was one of the biggest migrations in India in recent times and it posed a major challenge in implementation of the various welfare programmes, including the Government of India's TB Programme.

The government aims to achieve the UN's Sustainable Development Goal (SDG) of eliminating

TB by 2025 (the UN SDGs include ending the TB epidemic by 2030, under 'Goal'). It changed the name and logo of the TB Programme in 2020. The Revised National Tuberculosis Control Programme (RNTCP) was renamed the National Tuberculosis Elimination Programme (NTEP). A total of 14.75 lakh TB patients were notified under the Programme from January to October 2020, a decrease of 27% (20.28 lakh cases) as compared to the same period in 2019.

The Ministry of Health and Family Welfare attributes this to the impact of Covid-19 on TB services, repurposing of available resources and manpower, and restrictions imposed during the pandemic. About 36,514 Drug-resistant TB patients were notified during this period. The government has paid Rs 928.8 crore to 36.8 lakh TB patients under the Nikshay Poshan Yojana, towards nutritional support, from April 2018 to September 2020.[1]

While migrants were struggling to return to their home states, there was no mechanism in place even to ensure they had food and water. Indian states do not maintain proper records of migrant workers and tracking migrant TB patients has been an almost impossible task for the health machinery. But this is not just the impact of Covid-19; even in normal times, diagnosis and treatment of TB in migrant populations have remained a major challenge.

The National Framework for a Gender-Responsive Approach to TB in India, a report published by the Central TB Division, Ministry of Health and Family Welfare, highlights that it is difficult for migrants to adhere to treatment because of poor mechanisms to support uninterrupted treatment. Migrants face extreme poverty and are busy trying to earn a daily wage. This is more important for them than continuing TB treatment. When a migrant worker moves from one job or place to another, he/she discontinues treatment and does not provide a new work address as there is no permanent address. Also, there is no guarantee that he/she will work in the new place for a long period. Even if they have the address of their employer, migrants are unwilling to share it with the health system as they do not want to carry the stigma or lose employment because of the attached stigma. Migrants also do not have adequate identity proof.[2]

The WHO Note on Tuberculosis Prevention and Care for Migrants states that TB particularly affects poor and vulnerable populations; migrants are a key affected population. 'Migration as a social determinant of health increases TB-related morbidity and mortality for migrants and their communities along all migration pathways,' the Note states. It adds that migrants who have a legal status can access TB diagnosis and treatment, but this is subject to the work contracts they sign as well as their work permits. The ability of migrants to access healthcare services or insurance from the State or employer also plays a vital role in how TB is diagnosed and treated. Undocumented migrants—the majority of them in India fall into this category—fear losing their jobs and being sent back to their villages. This is a major hurdle in getting them access to diagnostic and treatment services.

'Deportation while on treatment or poor adherence may lead to drug-resistant disease, poor outcomes, and further spread of infection,' the WHO Note adds. Migrants living in detention centres or those who are trafficked face a worse situation. They live in unhealthy conditions for extended periods and create pockets of vulnerability to TB. 'Forced displacement of persons after conflict or a natural disaster is often associated with increased TB risk due to malnutrition, overcrowding in camps or other temporary shelters, treatment interruption from disruption of health services, and risk of drug resistance,' the WHO states.[3]

The Report of The Working Group on Migration by the Ministry of Housing and Urban Poverty Alleviation, published in 2017, reaffirms that migrants are exposed to health risks, including communicable diseases such as malaria and TB. They are also exposed to sexually transmitted diseases such as HIV, as well as occupational health hazards, including respiratory problems, lung diseases, allergies, kidney and bladder infections, back problems, and malnutrition. They are resultantly stigmatised as being carriers of disease.[4]

The 'TB Carrier'

Unable to pedal his tricycle rickshaw, Babu often used to step down and pull it. Often, his passengers would tell him that if he could not pedal the rickshaw, they would hail another one.

From morning till late night, Babu used to be on duty at the Mayur Vihar Extension metro railway station in New Delhi. He would only take a half-hour break for lunch. He continued this routine for almost a year. On most days, Babu would be the only rickshaw puller at the station when the last train came in. Many regular users of the metro knew him personally as he would always be waiting at the station, ready to ferry them home.

Babu's rickshaw was his home. Earlier, he used to live with a few labourers in a slum nearby, but he had to vacate the shared room as he could not contribute his share of the monthly rent. He was surviving by using public toilets and bathing by the roadside.

Babu had a swollen lymph node in his neck and the pain was unbearable. He had lost weight, but he continued to work since he had no other option.

Babu told people he belonged to a village near Muzaffarpur, Bihar. He was almost forty-five and wanted to return to his village after saving some money. But he was worried about how he would earn a living after returning. Babu had been getting treatment in his village for lymph node TB, but he had cut short the treatment and moved to New Delhi. It was not his first stint in the national capital. A few years earlier, he had gone to Delhi seeking work and was employed at a roadside dhaba (eatery). However, he had returned to his village within six months, finding it difficult to cope with life in the city. Subsequently, he had travelled to and from his village, Delhi, and Agra.

'Kaun apna gaon marji se chodta hai?' (Who leaves his village willingly?), he had asked me when I met him in 2018. As his neck pain increased, he procured painkillers from a doctor in Mayur Vihar. The doctor asked him to go for a further check-up to diagnose the lump, but Babu already knew that TB was the cause. He never revealed the past diagnosis to the doctor and instead took painkillers regularly.

By now, those who knew him suspected that the lump near his neck was cancerous. They repeatedly asked him to go to a cancer specialist. One day, Babu went missing from the metro station. Asked about his whereabouts, the other rickshaw drivers said that he had returned his rented rickshaw to the owner and left for his village.

Babu is just one of the millions of 'missing' TB patients in India. According to government data (National Strategic Plan for Tuberculosis Elimination: 2017-25), India has more than a million 'missing' cases every year that are not notified. Most remain undiagnosed or are unaccountably and inadequately diagnosed and treated in the private sector.

The Report of The Working Group on Migration states that the poor lack access to the healthcare system due to many factors. The private healthcare system is expensive. Migrants also have to take time off to make themselves available during the medical practitioners' hours of work. Most prefer to skip appointments and prioritise their own work as they do not want to lose out on their wages. Migrants also cannot afford to spend money on transportation to reach hospitals, which are often far away. Perceived alienation from government health systems at the destination and language difficulties also play a role in keeping them away from the healthcare system.[5]

The National Urban Health Mission Implementation Framework (NUHM) found that while the healthcare system in urban areas might be close to the poor, the poor may not be able to access the service because of the system's inadequacies, resulting in massive crowds seeking services. 'Ineffective outreach and a weak referral system also limit the access of urban poor to health care services. Social exclusion and lack of information and assistance at the secondary and tertiary hospitals make them unfamiliar to the modern environment of hospitals, thus restricting their access,' the NUHM framework adds.[6]

Who are Migrants?

In 2020, Union Minister for Agriculture and Farmers' Welfare Narendra Singh Tomar told the Lok Sabha during a discussion that the migration of agricultural labour from rural to urban India is a general phenomenon. The minister added that this was a natural part of the development process. 'The reasons for this shift include, inter alia, better employment opportunities in industry and services, increasing urbanization, low income in agriculture, etc. In a market economy like India, movement of the people for better economic opportunities is inexorable,' the Minister said. According to the Ministry of Finance, the Cohort-based Migration Metric (CMM) shows that inter-State labour mobility averaged 5-6.5 million people between 2001 and 2011, yielding an inter-State migrant population of about 60 million and inter-district migration as high as 80 million.[7]

Interestingly, despite all the challenges they face, migrants continue to flock to cities. An International Monetary Fund (IMF) research paper titled 'Inequality and Locational Determinants of the Distribution of Living Standards in India' by Sriram Balasubramanian,

Rishabh Kumar, and Prakash Loungani, has an interesting perspective on the issue. The paper says that an economic migrant (on average) expects a better life as a member of the lower class in a city compared to that of being in the middle class in a rural area. 'Given that rural India offers much lower living standards on average, a person may be indifferent to their relative class position and prefer the absolute gains emanating despite moving down in the class hierarchy,' the researchers observed. Using 2011-12 consumption micro-data, they found that nearly one-third of the variation in living standards in India can be explained by location alone.[8]

Back to Villages?

The researchers certainly have a point. Migrants in cities continue to live in pathetic conditions but are reluctant to go back to their villages. Slums thus become their homes. But the poor environmental conditions in the slums along with the high population density make them vulnerable to TB and other diseases. Slums also have a high incidence of vector-borne diseases (VBDs). Cases of malaria among the urban poor are twice as high as among other urban residents, according to the National Urban Health Mission Implementation Framework (NUHM).

According to the 2011 Census of India, a total of 6.54 crore people live in slums. The National

Sample Survey Office (NSSO), in its 69th Round on Urban Slums in India (2012), found that 33,510 slums exist in urban areas.

Anil Ghanwat, a farmer leader in Maharashtra, says that the majority of workers in the urban gig economy are small and marginal farmers or farm labourers who migrate to cities in search of a livelihood. 'Agriculture has been destroyed by the policies of consecutive governments and farmers are in distress. Farmers and farm labourers are moving to urban areas and living in slums. There are no job opportunities in rural areas and agriculture is not profit-making.' He opines that villagers should turn to agribusiness instead of sticking to traditional cultivation.

Maharashtra saw internal migration during the Covid-19 pandemic, with workers in Mumbai returning to their villages. Some of them have realised that there is no point in living in congested city slums and are innovating to survive and make farming profitable.

Koregaon, along with the Maan and Khatav tehsils, is one of the drought-prone regions of Maharashtra. For generations, the youth in these villages migrated to cities, especially Mumbai, to work as mathadi workers (head-loaders). They were not interested in farming, but the Covid-19 outbreak in Mumbai changed everything and there was a reverse migration to villages.

Over the last few years, farmers who chose to remain in Koregaon have toiled to cultivate strawberries using the available irrigation facilities and now, the new generation has joined them. Koregaon, a few kilometres from Mahabaleshwar, a hill station known for its strawberries, is emerging as another strawberry hub. The migrant youth who have returned have started digging wells to find a permanent solution to the chronic water scarcity in the region. Sharad Ingale, a farmer from Satara, says that living as a migrant is no less than living in hell. 'Forget proper food and health; you don't even get clean water to drink. We put our lives at risk while working in unhealthy conditions in cities. The slums in Mumbai are a den of TB,' he says.[9]

Like the youth in Koregaon, Babu and others like him would certainly prefer to stay home with their families if they are assured of a livelihood and a decent life. Unfortunately, Koregaon is an exception. And Babu and others like him remain a challenge for India's TB control programme. The massive migration to cities will continue to add to that challenge. Finding ways to motivate people to remain in their hometowns and villages is one of the biggest concerns Indian policymakers grapple with. Perhaps they can take some useful tips from the youth in Koregaon if they want to meaningfully address the problem.

NOTES

1. Ministry of Health and Family Welfare. (2020). Ministry of Health and Family Welfare 2020 Achievement. Retrieved from https://pib.gov.in/PressReleaseIframePage.aspx?PRID=1684546
2. Central TB Division, Ministry of Health and Family Welfare. (2019). National Framework for a Gender—Responsive approach to TB in India. Retrieved from—https://tbcindia.gov.in/WriteReadData/1892s/388838054811%20NTEP%20Gender%20Responsive%20Framework_311219.pdf
3. International Organization for Migration and World Health Organization. (2014). Tuberculosis Prevention and Care for Migrants. Retrieved from https://www.who.int/tb/publications/WHOIOM_TBmigration.pdf
4. Ministry of Housing and Urban Poverty Alleviation. (2017). Report of the Working Group on Migration. Retrieved from http://mohua.gov.in/upload/uploadfiles/files/1566.pdf
5. ibid.
6. Ministry of Health and Family Welfare. (2013). National Urban Health Mission. Retrieved from file:///D:/Users/11282/Desktop/TB%20Story/Stories/6.%20Migration/Implementation_Framework_NUHM.pdf
7. Jadhav, R. (2021). Five States account for 67% migrant workers who returned home during the lockdown. Retrieved from https://www.thehindubusinessline.

com/data-stories/data-focus/five-states-account-for-67-migrant-workers-who-returned-home-during-the-lockdown/article33813158.ece

8. Jadhav, R. (2021). Why location matters in determining living standards. Retrieved from https://www.thehindubusinessline.com/data-stories/data-focus/why-location-matters-in-determining-living-standards/article34029718.ece

9. Jadhav, R. (2020). Homeward bind: What lies ahead for migrants who have returned to Maharashtra's villages. Retrieved from https://www.thehindubusinessline.com/blink/cover/the-road-ahead-for-migrants-who-have-returned-to-their-villages-in-maharashtra/article31921469.ece

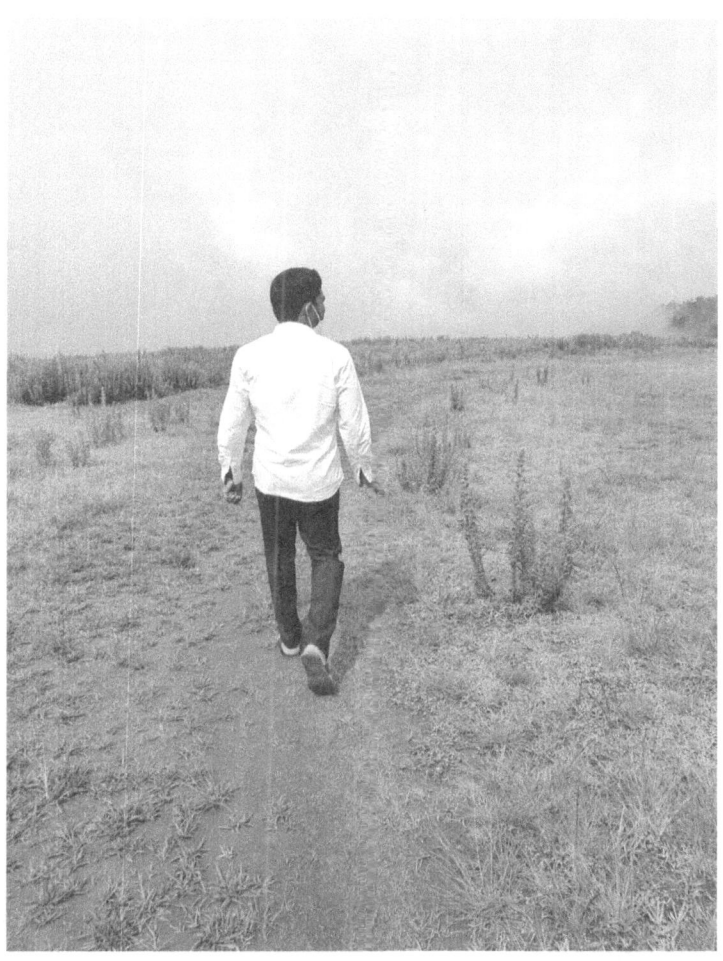

For many TB patients, their families, and close friends, life becomes a lonely battle as they face boycott from society. *(picture credit: Radheshyam Jadhav)*

11

Stigma and TB: Myths and Reality

Sixty-year-old Ramnath's (name changed on request) life took an unimaginable turn. He had become a pariah in his own house. His family members, including his young children, wanted him to leave the house and live separately. By dint of his hard work, Ramnath, a farmer, had sustained his family through the agrarian crises that wracked the region. The vagaries of nature have affected farming in Beed district, a part of the Marathwada region, which has become infamous as a farmer-suicide zone.

Ramnath had managed to fend off the horrors that accompanied drought, but now he found himself defenceless and devastated. His family wanted to ostracise him because he had been diagnosed with TB. They warned him against sharing the news with relatives and neighbours. Ramnath began his treatment at a Primary Health Centre (PHC). Doctors told him that the TB was curable and that he would completely recover.

Ramnath told his family that with the proper treatment he would be back to normal, but they were not willing to believe this. Very disturbed, he left the house. To his chagrin, nobody asked him to stay or bothered to bring him back. In the end, he returned home on his own. He was a habitual drinker and had started consuming more alcohol after he was diagnosed with TB.

Ramnath was not worried about how the world would react to his TB diagnosis. But he was hurt by the behaviour of his family and that of the villagers. He cursed himself for contracting TB and took a drastic decision. He stopped his treatment saying that he did not want to live anymore. His family had always been his first priority and he had sacrificed everything for them. But now that they had rejected him, at a time when he needed them the most, he had no desire to live. One of his sons is a driver in Mumbai while the other is a farmer in the village. Neither supported him.

Even the government health system was not enthusiastic about his treatment as he was written off as a 'drunkard'.

'The government is making a great deal of effort

to identify TB patients and ASHA workers are doing a great job. Ramnath's case was detected during a check-up in the village,' says the husband of an ASHA worker in the locality. Initially, the ASHA worker was not willing to speak, and her husband had to do all the talking over the phone.

Asked to elaborate on Ramnath's case, the ASHA worker says, 'We have asked him to eat eggs and meat. And he has recovered. But he continues to drink.' The husband pipes in from the background saying, 'There is no point in meeting him. He starts drinking in the morning and has lost his senses.' The husband then takes over the conversation saying that his wife has to attend an urgent meeting.

'He is not at home. He is away in the field. I can't tell you when you can meet him,' says Ramnath's son, when asked about his father. He fears that an outsider coming to the small village and that, too, to meet his father, would attract unwanted attention. He hints that normalcy has just begun to return to the family after Ramnath's bout with TB. The son is unwilling to talk about his father's disease or his alcoholism.

The health machinery was happy to add another case to its tally and move closer to its TB diagnosis target. But for Ramnath, life is very difficult. Whenever he steps out of the house, people avoid him. When he is at the temple, people literally run away to avoid contact with him.

There are hundreds and thousands of TB patients facing Ramnath's predicament. The National Family Health Survey (NFHS-4) observed that TB is a curable disease but can be stigmatising, mainly due to people's ignorance of its etiology and transmission. The survey has some interesting data. 87% of women aged 15-49 and 88% of men aged 15-49 have heard of TB. Of these, 69% of women and 72% of men are aware that coughing or sneezing are modes of transmission of the disease. But more than half the population that has heard of TB has some misconceptions regarding its transmission. The survey adds that one in every six women and one in every five men report they would want the TB positive status of a family member to remain a secret. 89% of women and 91% of men who have heard of TB believe that it can be cured, according to the survey.

NFHS-4 highlights that the proportion of women who have heard of TB generally increases steadily with the level of schooling and the wealth index, from about four-fifths of women in the lowest schooling and wealth categories to well over 90% in the highest schooling and wealth categories. The pattern of schooling and wealth levels is the same for men, as far as TB awareness is concerned.

TB has re-emerged as a major public health problem in many parts of the world, often as a concomitant illness to HIV/AIDS. The survey states that TB was once known as the 'white plague' and would continue to be a serious health threat even in the absence of HIV/AIDS due to the public health challenges posed by poor sanitation, poverty, and high illiteracy.[1]

What is it All About?

TB and research on it in India go back to 1906, when a Christian organization in Ajmer district established the first open-air sanitorium. In 1929, India joined the International Union Against Tuberculosis (IUAT). According to a WHO document on the history of tuberculosis control in India, The King George V Thanks Giving Fund for TB control was established and administered through central, state, and provincial committees to support TB education and prevention, establish clinics, and train health workers. In 1939, the TB Association of India (TAI) was established to develop standard methods to manage TB and develop model training institutions.[2]

But for the thousands like Ramnath and his family, TB is still a myth and a stigma. As with many other diseases, a big chunk of the educated and uneducated masses in India still believes that TB is caused by a divine curse or due to heredity. The fact is, TB is caused by the bacterium Mycobacterium tuberculosis and most often affects the lungs. It spreads through the air when people with lung TB cough, sneeze or spit. The infection passes to a person if he/she inhales just a few germs, according to the WHO. However, the WHO also states that TB is preventable and that it can be cured using antibiotics. Every year, ten million people fall ill with TB worldwide and 1.5 million people die, with over 95% of the cases and deaths occurring in developing countries. TB tops the infectious diseases chart and is the leading cause of death of people with HIV. It is also a major contributor to antimicrobial resistance.

The WHO has noted that TB has spread its tentacles across the world, but most of those who contract the disease are from low and middle-income countries. India, along with Bangladesh, China, Indonesia, Nigeria, Pakistan, the Philippines, and South Africa, is home to half of all people with TB. One quarter of the world's population is estimated to be infected with TB bacteria and about 5-15% fall ill with active TB. While the rest carry the TB bacteria, they do not fall ill and cannot transmit the disease. TB mostly affects adults in their most productive years, though all age groups are at risk. Those who suffer from other conditions that impair the immune system face an active TB risk. Alcohol abuse and smoking increase the risk of contracting TB by a factor of 3.3 and 1.6, respectively. In 2019, 0.72 million new TB cases worldwide were attributable to alcohol use and 0.70 million were attributable to smoking.[3]

Survivors Against TB (SATB) explains it well. TB can affect any part of the body and it can be divided into two categories. The first category is pulmonary TB, which impacts the lungs. This most common TB is infectious and could spread through coughing/sneezing. The second category is extra-pulmonary TB or EPTB, which impacts other body parts. It is not infectious and is relatively less common. Once inside the body, it can spread through the blood or lymphatic system to different organs and body parts such as lymph nodes, brain, spine, bone, etc. Sometimes, TB can be disseminated and involve multiple organs at the same time.

'Some typical symptoms of pulmonary TB include low fever for a prolonged duration (3-4 hours) and especially in the evening; weight loss; loss of appetite; prolonged cough (for more than two weeks); coughing blood; and night sweats. Apart from the symptoms mentioned above, symptoms of extra-pulmonary TB include severe localised pain (in the area that may be affected by EPTB),' says SATB.[4]

The efforts of international agencies, governments, and NGOs working to eradicate TB notwithstanding, myths and misconceptions continue to prevail among the majority of the people.

Myths and Stigma

Ramnath's sons fear that since their father has TB, they, too, will contract it and that every generation in the family will have to battle the disease. Fear of death makes TB even more lethal in the minds of the masses and many believe that a TB patient will have HIV or vice versa. Also, there is a fear of TB causing infertility and impotency.

The Strategy to End Stigma and Discrimination Associated with Tuberculosis, by the Central TB Division of the Ministry of Health and Family Welfare, notes that stigma arises out of fear of TB. It is also related to health, financial conditions, and the social consequences TB has on patients and their families. 'Stigma exacerbates the medical and social hardships of TB and is responsible for delays in diagnosis and treatment initiation, treatment interruptions, and poor outcomes. Stigma is a barrier to TB elimination,' states the strategy document. It adds, 'Stigma is a phenomenon whereby an individual with an attribute that is deeply discredited by his/her society is rejected as a result of that attribute.' Stigma is a process where an individual is disqualified from full social acceptance as a reaction to TB. The WHO defines stigma as a mark of shame, disgrace or disapproval, which results in an individual being rejected, discriminated against, and excluded from participating in a number of different activities in society.[5]

'Misconceptions and stigma are major hurdles in dealing with TB cases. The government has failed on this front. But one cannot blame the government alone. We as a society are not able to grow mature. The way we react and respond to diseases like TB is a reflection of our overall character as a society. Ramnath's case, which I have seen personally, is an example of how we handle TB,' said a medical practitioner who works with the Indian Council of Medical Research (ICMR), handling TB and Covid-19-related research. He added that TB still remains a taboo that many people are not willing to speak about or acknowledge.

Survivors Show the Way

SATB, a community-based movement, is the exception. This community comprises TB survivors, who share their experiences on various platforms. Their stories have helped many TB patients deal with TB and the resultant stigma and discrimination. 'SATB believes that if India wishes to address TB comprehensively, it needs to start by listening to survivors and engaging them in policy-making that affects them the most,' the SATB website declares, with the faces of confident and brave survivors dotting the home page.

Deepti Chavan, a patient advocate and multidrug-resistant TB (MDR-TB) survivor, says that people tried to dissuade her when she wanted to speak about TB. Deepti was determined to communicate her six-year experience. At the age of sixteen, when she was preparing for her board exams, she was diagnosed with TB and later with MDR-TB. Today, Deepti has become a supportive voice for all those undergoing treatment. Saurabh Rane, a development professional and MDR-TB survivor, identifies lack of awareness and family support, misdiagnosis, expensive treatment, poor nutrition, and absence of counselling as the problems most patients face. People must be empowered with information and awareness, he insists. Arun Singh Rana, a public health professional, shares his and his father's story, highlighting the need for accurate diagnosis of the disease.

Debshree Lokhande, an architect who is an extremely drug-resistant TB (XXDR-TB) survivor, is a committed, outspoken, and fearless advocate who shares her experiences so that people become aware about the facts of the disease. Debshree talks of people, uninformed medical practitioners, and friends who left her all alone in her battle. Many TB patients would easily identify with her experience. Himanshu Patel and Diptendu Bhattacharya—both MDR-TB survivors, open up about their story of struggle and hope without any qualms.

Sandhya Krishnan, a wellness coach and TB survivor, has learned a lesson that she shares with others: good nutrition and wellness are essential to prevent a plethora of diseases. 'TB is curable. Let us collectively fight against it. The right diagnosis, proper treatment, and much-needed awareness about it are necessary to defeat TB. We must fight against TB, not those affected by it,' declares Keyuri Bhanushali, a copywriter and MDR-TB survivor. Manasi Khade, a photographer and an extensively drug-resistant TB (XDR-TB) survivor, tells her gritty story and talks about the way she dealt with the disease. MBA student Ritu Khattar, another TB survivor, says, 'The battle with TB and its side-effects has been extremely challenging, but each failure and each moment of being bullied and put down by people have made me stronger.'

Ashna Ashesh, an MDR-TB survivor, patient advocate, and lawyer, found TB physically and emotionally consuming. Bulbul Sharma, a teacher and TB survivor, says, 'The experience altered my life. It has changed me for good and has strengthened my relationship with my family. I am more patient, have a higher tolerance for things going wrong, empathetic, and probably the best version of myself.'

These survivors with SATB are torchbearers, and their stories will encourage TB patients and their families and friends to shed the stigma and misconceptions around the disease. Survivors who have fought and triumphed over TB are probably the best messengers to turn the tide against the inhuman treatment and discrimination that so many patients in India face.[6]

NOTES

1. Ministry of Health and Family Welfare. (2015-16). National Family Health Survey 2015-16. Retrieved from http://rchiips.org/nfhs/nfhs-4Reports/India.pdf
2. World Health Organization. (2010). A brief history of tuberculosis control in India. Retrieved from http://apps.who.int/iris/bitstream/handle/10665/44408/9789241500159_eng.pdf,jsessionid=555DF65AD68BF4092140C671F3F51B21?sequence=1
3. World Health Organization. (2020). Tuberculosis. Retrieved from https://www.who.int/news-room/fact-sheets/detail/tuberculosis
4. Survivors Against TB. (2021). Frequently Asked Questions. Retrieved from https://survivorsagainsttb.com/En/faq.php
5. Central TB Division, Ministry of Health and Family Welfare. (2021). Strategy to End Stigma and Discrimination Associated with Tuberculosis. Retrieved from https://tbcindia.gov.in/WriteReadData/l892s/2581521802 Strategy%20to%20End%20Stigma%20and%20Discrimination%20Associated%20with% 20TB%2018032021%20New.pdf
6. Survivors Against TB. (2021). Our Survivors. Retrieved from https://survivorsagainsttb.com/En/survivor.php

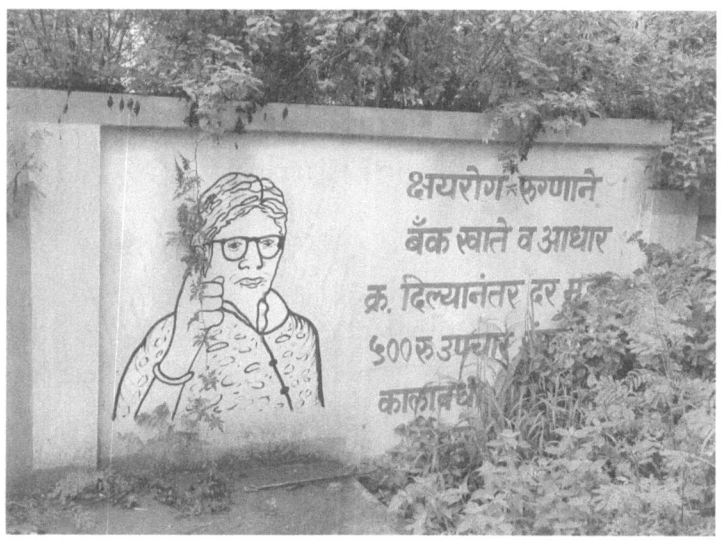

TB patients from poor families faced a dual challenge throughout the Covid-19 pandemic, but Rs 500 per month given by the government for TB treatment helped them to survive. The government is highlighting this assistance in advertisements. *(picture credit: Radheshyam Jadhav)*

12

Covid-19 Pandemic and TB: A Dual Burden

Saubai and many other elder villagers in the small town of Beed were completely shaken by what was happening around them. The news channels were displaying piles of dead bodies of Covid-19 patients and the newspapers were full of similar news and pictures.

The WHO country office in India alerted the Central government on 6th January 2020 about the outbreak of pneumonia of unknown origin in the city of Wuhan, China. The WHO issued a statement on 9th January 2020, about a novel coronavirus. It was later named SARS-CoV-2, and the disease it caused was called Covid-19 by the WHO on 11th February 2020. The first Indian case of Covid-19 was reported on 30th January 2020, and from March 2020, a series of lockdowns began, continuing into 2021.[1]

Saubai was so shocked by the Covid-19 news and discussions all around that she stopped going out to socialise. She feared that if she contracted Covid-19 she would not be able to recover and would die an isolated death. Images of bodies wrapped in plastic bags handled by health workers haunted her and others. Her husband, two sons, and daughters-in-law tried to comfort her in every possible way, but she was filled with extreme fear. One day, she had a cough and broke down, refusing to avail any treatment. It took the family a great deal of effort to get her to go for a Covid-19 test. While waiting for the test result, she prayed all day and refused to eat.

'The Covid-19 test was negative and she was relieved. She was happy that her cough was nothing but a normal one and would go away with cough syrup. We started medication for the cough. But instead of improving, it kept getting worse and we were confused,' says her son, who runs a stationery shop. With Saubai's cough not responding to any treatment, her elder son began to suspect she had TB. About ten years earlier, his brother, who is in Mumbai, had contracted TB.

'But my brother had recovered completely. I decided to take my mother to the Primary Health Centre (PHC) for TB tests but didn't tell her about it. I told her that we needed to get some routine tests done for her cough. She was not ready to come to the hospital, but I told her that a continuous cough is not a good sign, especially during the Covid-19 pandemic. Her TB was confirmed after tests. But I told her that the reports were normal,' her son added.

Saubai's treatment commenced. She was shifted to another room in the house and family members started wearing masks within the house. She realised that something was wrong and asked why so many tablets were being given to her and why she was being isolated when she was not a Covid-19 patient.

The family members decided that she must not be kept in the dark and told her about the TB diagnosis. Saubai was shocked. She said that TB had come as a stigma in the last stage of her life. 'Please don't tell anyone about this,' she implored family members, tearfully blaming her destiny for the disease.

'She will not speak to anyone,' said her husband, when I requested a meeting with her. 'She has strictly said that her TB diagnosis should not be revealed to anyone. We are somehow trying to bring her confidence back. And you media people will create unnecessary problems.'

Saubai was fortunate to have family support, which is not the case for many patients. 'Diagnosing TB almost stopped during the first phase of the Covid wave and it took a lot of time for the health machinery to realise that TB patients are being neglected while paying attention to Covid-19. In rural areas, the situation was worse as the health infrastructure and manpower is very limited,' a government health official monitoring the TB programme in rural areas of Maharashtra admitted.

The Government of India came out with a Rapid Response Plan to mitigate the impact of the Covid pandemic on the TB Epidemic and National TB Elimination Programme (NTEP) activities in India. According to this plan, lockdowns during the Covid pandemic affected all the key strategic interventions, resulting in an almost 60% decline in TB notification. This resulted in a regression to the time when the gap between estimated TB cases and notified TB cases was increasing. TB is an infectious bacterial disease. It primarily targets the lungs and is transmitted through droplet nuclei. 'One pulmonary TB patient, if untreated, can infect 10-15 individuals in a year. In such circumstances, when TB patients are not able to access health services and are confined within their homes, there is all likelihood of active intense transmission in the household contacts,' states the Rapid Response Plan document.

Lack of medical attention leads to significant morbidity among TB patients. Lockdowns could lead to TB-related deaths due to non-diagnosis/no treatment/discontinuation of anti-TB medication.

'Recent modelling studies to understand the potential effect of the Covid-19 response on TB epidemiology published by Stop TB Partnership indicates that over and above the existing cases, there would be an additional 5,14,370 TB cases and 1,51,120 TB deaths over the next five years,' the document adds.[2]

Shattered Rural Economy

Santaji (name changed), a young TB patient from Nashik who works as a farm labourer, has had to face a dual challenge through the Covid-19 pandemic. He was diagnosed with TB, and at the same time, he lost work due to the lockdown. 'Though the government said that agricultural activities would continue, everything was at a standstill. Already, I had lost weight and was not able to work continuously. But the lockdown deprived me of whatever work I was getting,' he says. Under the government's Nikshay Poshan Yojana (NPY), Santaji gets Rs 500 for each month of treatment. The objective of the government is to provide nutritional support to TB patients at the time of notification and subsequently during the course of their treatment.

'So, what nutritional food do you eat using this money?'

'I eat nutritional food,' is all he will say, squirming in his chair in the Primary Health Centre. Prodded for a response, he has a counter-question, 'Will the government stop giving me money if it finds out that I don't eat nutritional food using this money?' During the lockdown, Santaji's only income was this Rs 500 and his family somehow survived on the money.

Covid-19-induced lockdowns and financial distress disturbed the fabric of rural life. The number of workers under the Mahatma Gandhi National Rural Employment Guarantee Scheme (MGNREGS) is an indication of how the rural economy came under intense stress. The welfare scheme tries to enhance the livelihood security by providing at least 100 days of guaranteed wage employment in every financial year to every household whose adult members volunteer to do unskilled manual work.

During financial year 2020-21, a total of 1.89 crore new job cards were issued under MGNREGS and the total number of job cards issued by August 2021-22 stood at 56.47 lakh. During 2020-21, a total of 389 crore persondays were generated, which is 47% more than the previous financial year. In 2020-21, a total of 7.55 crore households were provided employment, 38% more than in the previous financial year.[3]

Poor and unorganized-sector workers suffered the most during the pandemic. In India, the wages of formal workers were cut by 3.6%, while informal workers experienced a much sharper fall in wages, at 22.6%, during the Covid-induced lockdown, the International Labour Organization's (ILO) Global Wage Report noted. The report estimated that 40 lakh and 6.94 crore informally employed workers were at risk of losing their jobs during lockdown 1.0 and lockdown 2.0, respectively. Informally employed workers in the unorganized sector suffered wage losses amounting to Rs 63,553 crore (Rs 635.53 billion).[4]

TB Cases to Covid-19

In July 2021, the Ministry of Health and Family Welfare issued a statement on media reports alleging a sudden rise in TB cases among patients who were infected with Covid-19, with worried doctors reportedly seeing around a dozen such cases every day.

'It is clarified that tuberculosis (TB) screening for all Covid-19 positive patients and Covid-19 screening for all diagnosed TB patients has been recommended by the Ministry of Health and Family Welfare. States/UTs have been asked for convergence in efforts for better surveillance and case finding of TB and Covid-19, as early as August 2020,' the Ministry stated.

The Ministry added that due to the impact of Covid-19-related restrictions, case notifications for TB had decreased by about 25% in 2020, but special efforts were being made to mitigate this impact through intensified case detection in OPD settings as well as through active case finding campaigns within the community by all States.

Helping Hand

'Covid-19 has made us rethink our social, political, and economic priorities. It has exposed us to the vulnerability of life. I hope that we become more human and more rational when we deal with the poor suffering from TB or any other disease. Of course, this is just hope. But what we can do at our level we must start doing immediately without waiting for others to take action,' says Aniket Lohiya of Ambajogai who runs the Beed district-based organization Manavlok. The organization's community kitchens for elderly villagers have proved to be life-savers for rural residents during the pandemic. Free community dining houses called Trupti Kitchens provide two nutritious fresh meals per day to senior villagers, while village committees also provide medicines, clothing, shelter, and other necessities.[6]

For sixty-year-old ragpicker Gawalanbai Ujagare, every single rupee is as precious as a thousand as she earns just Rs 6,000 per month. Gawalanbai, who lives in Pune, felt that her country needed her help in the fight against the virus. She donated her hard-earned savings of Rs 15,000 to the Chief Minister's relief fund during the pandemic. There was a simple rationale driving her action—it does not matter if you are poor or rich. What matters is your intention and will to help others.

'During the Covid-19 pandemic, every person who was infected must have realised what it means to be boycotted and discriminated against. Like TB, Covid doesn't discriminate between poor or rich, educated or uneducated...We must try to become human beings. When you target a TB patient by treating her in an inhuman way, imagine yourself and your loved ones in the shoes of a TB patient,' says Sunanda (also known as Rupali Bhanuse), who has fought TB and is fighting HIV. She adds that while every TB patient must hope for better treatment from society, at the end of the day it is a battle each individual has to fight on his/her own, with grit and determination.

NOTES

1. Ministry of Health and Family Welfare. (2020). Assessment of Covid Prevention. Retrieved from https://pib.gov.in/PressReleaseIframePage.aspx?PRID=1656184
2. Ministry of Health and Family Welfare. (2020). Rapid Response Plan to mitigate impact of COVID-19 Pandemic on TB Epidemic and National TB Elimination Programme (NTEP). Retrieved from https://tbcindia.gov.in/WriteReadData/l892s/60159559755DODDG_NTEP%20Rapid%20Response_Full.pdf
3. Jadhav, R. (2021). How MGNREGS turned lifeline for rural India during the pandemic. Retrieved from https://www.thehindubusinessline.com/data-stories/data-focus/how-mgnregs-turned-lifeline-for-rural-india-during-the-pandemic/article35854703.ece
4. Jadhav, R. (2021). Covid-19: How much did unorganised sector lose? Retrieved from https://www.thehindubusinessline.com/economy/covid-19-lockdowns-how-much-did-the-unorganised-sector-lose/article33491316.ece
5. Ministry of Health and Family Welfare. (2021). COVID19: Myths vs. Facts. Retrieved from https://pib.gov.in/PressReleseDetailm.aspx?PRID=1736417
6. Jadhav, R. (2021). Covid-19: How the community managed kitchens to feed elderly rural folk. Retrieved from https://www.thehindubusinessline.com/news/national/covid-19-how-the-community-managed-kitchens-to-feed-elderly-rural-folk/article35403933.ece

Annexure

FREQUENTLY ASKED QUESTIONS (FAQs) ABOUT TB

Does TB only affect the lungs? Which other parts of the body can the bacteria affect?

Tuberculosis can affect any part of the body. But it can be categorized into two broad categories:

1. Pulmonary TB (impacts the lungs). This type is infectious. It spreads through the acts of coughing/sneezing and is more common.

2. Extra-Pulmonary TB or EPTB (impacts other body parts than the lungs). This type is not infectious to others and is relatively less common.

In most cases, the person is infected by the simple act of breathing around a person with active disease. Once inside the body, it can spread through the blood or the lymphatic system to different organs/body parts (such as lymph node, brain, spine, bone, etc.). Sometimes, TB can be disseminated and can involve multiple organs at the same time.

What is the most common symptom of TB?

Some typical symptoms of pulmonary TB include: low fever for a prolonged duration (3-4 hours), especially in the evening; weight loss; loss of appetite; prolonged cough (for more than two weeks); coughing blood; and night sweats. Apart from the symptoms mentioned above, symptoms of extra-pulmonary TB (EPTB) include severe localized pain (area which may be affected by EPTB). It is advised that family members wear masks at all times.

Have I been diagnosed correctly and given the right medication?

Every condition is unique and would require a medically qualified individual to confirm the diagnosis and verify the treatment. However, if drug sensitivity testing (DST) is conducted, it would be clearer which medicines will work, and which will not. DST should be done mandatorily. Moreover, if you wish to take a second opinion for mental satisfaction, never hesitate to take one from a qualified specialist.

What tests are to be done to confirm the diagnosis?

Basic sputum tests, X-ray, and drug sensitivity testing are performed to confirm the diagnosis and treatment status. In other cases, CT, Sonography, FNAC, etc. might be required.

How long will I have to undergo treatment? I have already been taking medicines for a year or so.

TB treatment is determined by the kind of TB you have. It can vary from a period of six months to two years or more. TB treatment should be monitored by a doctor and can only be stopped once the doctor gives approval after all the tests have been done. If one stops the treatment prior to a doctor's approval, it can lead to complications. For treatment, caution must be exercised and all decisions must be made with the doctor's permission.

What is the difference between types of TB? Why am I being given different medicines now? Why was I given different medicines before?

TB bacteria can manifest in different forms. If the bacterium attacks the lungs, it is called pulmonary TB and if it attacks other body parts (spleen, spine, stomach, etc.) it is known as extra-pulmonary TB (EPTB). Both the forms of TB can also manifest as drug-resistant. The variation in the prescription of medication is dependent on the kind of TB you have, the degree of drug-resistance, as well as the phase of treatment you may be in.

Are injections necessary?

Injectables are an integral part of second line TB treatment when a patient fails the first line treatment, i.e., treatment for multidrug-resistant TB (MDR-TB).

As one progresses from one form of drug-resistance to another, the treatment changes and injectables are included to cure severe forms of drug-resistance.

Is it completely curable or will I have to keep coming back after my treatment is done?

TB is completely curable provided the disease is diagnosed accurately; appropriate treatment is administered, and one completes the course of the treatment. One should visit the designated government centres to avail free diagnosis and treatment. Once declared TB free, one can lead a normal life coupled with a healthy, nutritious diet.

How do I get my medicines for free? My doctor is in Delhi, and I am from Lucknow.

You will have to enrol yourself in a TB programme at any government hospital. You can get your medicines for free from there. There is a government helpline as well that you can call.

How does the spacing for medicines happen?

Spacing between medicines is different for different conditions. It also varies depending upon the dosage and the type of medicine that you are consuming. You doctor is best suited to advise you on it.

What side-effects will the medicines cause?

TB medicines and especially drug-resistant TB medicines cause a variety of side-effects. These include nausea, severe headaches, and tiredness. These depend on the medication one is taking. However, these side-effects can be addressed, if you speak to the doctor about it. In more severe forms of TB, the side-effects can include partial blindness, hearing impairment, ocular complaints as well as impact on the heart. This, however, is restricted to the most extreme cases only.

In all cases, your effort should be to be vigilant and careful. You must create a log of side-effects so that you can monitor these and report these to the doctor when you visit him/her.

What do I do when I suffer from side-effects like vomiting and neuropathy?

Vomiting is a very common effect and causes weakness. Adequate hydration along with a balanced diet is essential to keep the body stable. Not just that, but small measures like sitting up straight after meals, eating shorter meals every two hours, and using antacid or ENO after taking the doctor's permission might also prove helpful.

Neuropathy is a side-effect that needs to be reported to the doctor immediately to take necessary steps. Loss of sensation, reduced vision, difficulty in hearing, etc. should be reported at the earliest to the doctor. In all cases, your effort should be to be vigilant and careful. You must create a log of side-effects so that you can monitor these and report these to the doctor when you go and see him/her.

I can't keep medicines down because of vomiting, so should I take the dose again?

If vomiting happens after the medicine is taken, it might not be necessary. But if it happens during intake, or if the medicine is also vomited, most likely it would have to be consumed again. It is best to check with the doctor for this, and also consider asking if tablets can be crushed and consumed if needed.

How do I know if the side-effects have started? Are there any tests to be done from time to time?

Most side-effects are minor and transient in nature. But sometimes, major side-effects like recurrent vomiting, vision/hearing problems, neuropathy, severe drug allergies, etc. can occur. These must be reported to the doctor and correctional measures should be taken.

Ideally, routine investigations like complete blood count (CBC), liver function test, kidney function test, blood sugar, thyroid levels, etc. should be done and repeated monthly or as per the doctor's orders. In some cases, specialized tests like audiometry, vision test, retina check, etc. need to be done too.

Repeating such investigations regularly can detect most adverse effects at the early stages and enable your doctor to take necessary correctional measures.

When will the vomiting and dizziness stop?

This may vary by body type and is dependent on the time taken by the body to get attuned to the medicines. However, it is important to be patient and recognise that these side-effects do eventually disappear. Keep your doctor updated on the side-effects such that remedial action can be taken, if required.

How did you cope with side-effects, especially reduced hearing and partial blindness?

A positive outlook towards life helped me immensely. I assured myself that the side-effects will disappear soon and I just have to bear them for a few days. Actually, I was out of options. I knew that I had to get well, and I will have to battle the side-effects. However, I did tell my doctor about them and saw a specialist too to mitigate doubts.

Can any of the TB medicines cause depression? If so, how does one deal with it?

Depression is a common side-effect of TB medication. One must be prepared for it. This is only possible through counselling, which entails preparing the patient for the side-effects of the medicines as well as providing support all through the treatment. Additionally, the patient must cooperate with the counsellor and keep him/her up-to-date about all side-effects. This will put in place a clear communication channel between the counsellor and the patient, which is key to effective therapy and in turn, TB treatment. If your doctor is unable to provide counselling please contact SATB with your questions and queries.

Will the buzzing/ringing sound in my ear continue for life?

Spot the lack of hearing in time/get tested for it every 2-3 months depending on your doctor's advice. Be aware that any reduction in hearing should be brought to the doctor's notice immediately.

Most women ask if they would be able to conceive after the completion of treatment.

Conception is dependent on a variety of factors, including hormonal balance and health of the uterus, amongst others. The most suitable and conclusive advice for this can come from your medical practitioner after tests and adequate check-ups. In some cases, there is a possibility that one may not be able to conceive after TB (especially if TB affects the uterus), however, with technology advancing in leaps and bounds, a number of methods have surfaced to help women conceive.

Should I maintain a high-protein diet even after completion of treatment?

Yes, one should maintain a balanced, protein-enriched diet, and a healthy lifestyle even after one's treatment ends.

Since pulmonary TB is communicable, what precautions should family members take?

Family members must wear masks at all times. Cross-ventilation and sunlight must be ensured to cut down on transmission. Everyone, including the patient, must consume a healthy diet to maintain immunity. This way, the patient can recover faster and the family can avoid getting infected.

Should one wear a mask in order to not infect anyone?

If your doctor has declared you to be non-infectious, there is no need to wear a mask. However, since

TB takes a deep toll on the immune system, even if you are non-infectious, continue to wear a mask as a way to protect yourself. Many believe masks lead to loss of self-confidence and of course stigma. Needless to say, if you are still being treated and are infectious, wear a mask at all times in order to not infect others.

How will TB affect my physical intimacy with my partner if one of us has TB?

Physical intimacy is different for everyone, but it is the nature of the act as well as the nature of diagnosis that determine if it is safe for you and your partner. Kissing, for example, may lead to infection/transmission more commonly in the case of pulmonary TB.

While sexual transmission of TB is rare, it has been noted considerably in medical literature. The chances of transmission are further reduced if the infected person is on treatment and the partner has strong immunity. If sexual transmission occurs, the disease may affect the reproductive organs and lead to reproductive problems later. Individuals with genital tuberculosis might transmit the disease through sexual contact. Before you engage in any such activity, it is best you consult a doctor and discuss your options and doubts thoroughly.

What diet should one follow?

A balanced diet comprising an optimum mix of protein and carbohydrates is essential to sustain TB treatment. Additionally, green leafy vegetables, eggs, bananas, vitamins, and minerals help to boost the immune system. It is important to make a diet chart if you can and ask for your doctor's inputs so that you can monitor your diet.

Will I need surgery?

The decision about surgery rests with the physician. Typically, surgery is considered the last resort.

What exercises should one do? How do they help?

One should opt for strolls or pranayama (breathing exercise). The process of recovery is slow but one has to realise that exercise is critical once recovery begins. This helps build immunity and also keeps one's spirits up.

When were you able to ambulate and work?

My case was very difficult so it took years for me to return to my normal routine. However, this is something you can eventually achieve. The key is having a positive attitude. Many people try and work part time and then slowly move on to full-time work to ensure that they keep up with their careers. Also, continue reading and updating your skills while you cannot work. This is very important.

How do I find work? My office says I can't work from home anymore because it's been quite some time.

You can request your doctor to write a letter to your organization explaining your condition. If you do not want that, then you can look for new part-time employment.

Does TB put a fullstop to one's dreams and ambitions?

TB is a perfectly curable disease. The trick lies in early, quick, and accurate diagnosis coupled with uninterrupted treatment. If either of these components are not adhered to, TB can be fatal. TB-affected individuals can achieve anything post treatment.

Private or government sector: which care is better?

While both entities offer TB services, it is the public sector (government) which provides free diagnosis and treatment services. The challenge with the private sector is that it offers erratic prescription practices as well as inaccurate diagnostic services, which perpetuate the transmission of drug-resistant TB.

However, to its advantage, the private sector offers confidentiality, hospitality as well as proximity.

How do I enrol for the government's TB programme?

Call the government's toll-free helpline to ask for details about enrolling in the TB programme. Or go to the nearest government dispensary to ask for the same. Alternatively, you can get yourself registered at a local government hospital. If you would like confidentiality, please ensure that the drugs are delivered by the DOTS provider at your home.

Will the disease affect one's chances of marriage?

The deep-seated stigma associated with TB is a significant issue but the disease does not affect the chances of marriage at all. It is all in the minds of the people who interact with you.

Is there a reason to panic if one's menstruation cycle becomes irregular or stops?

Disruption in the menstrual cycle is dependent on several factors, including hormonal imbalance. If the delay in periods is persistent, then one must consult the doctor before going ahead with any medication. Self-medication is strongly discouraged as drug interaction may lead to further damage. Always inform your doctor before you decide to pop that pill.

I'm waiting for my fever to subside. When will I have enough energy to walk and do my job?

It takes time for one's body to adjust to the medicine. As soon as medicines start working, the severity of symptoms will reduce, one will start to feel hungry again and the fever will also subside. However, one needs to give time for the treatment to show affect. Treatment needs to be completed, irrespective of how one feels. It is important to keep busy and upbeat. Think positive, express gratitude for small joys. The road to recovery becomes less stressful then.

What is the correlation between TB, poverty, and nutrition in India?

TB in particular affects a large number of India's poor due to social, economic, and environmental factors. Of these, poverty and undernutrition are well-established risk factors for TB in the country. Evidence has shown that both these factors are directly linked to completing TB treatment and its recovery. People with TB frequently experience severe economic barriers to health care, including high expenses related to diagnosis and treatment, as well as indirect costs due to loss of income. This is particularly true of those who work in the informal sector. Poor nutrition is inextricably linked to poverty and hunger. It delays recovery and also causes higher mortality among those who are affected by TB.

How does the economic burden due to TB affect the poor?

For the poor, the economic burden of TB creates barriers to prompt diagnosis, which may then lead to continuing transmission. When diagnosed, expenses such as transportation and the cost of food, combined with the loss of income, push families into debt and are disincentives to continuing treatment. A study established that an individual diagnosed with TB in India loses an average of three months' worth of wages. Delayed, interrupted, and incomplete treatment due to poverty not only poses a serious risk to individual health, but also increases the disease risk to others in the household and beyond. Poor nutrition among the TB-infected leads to wasting, poor recovery, and often unsuccessful treatment outcomes. For poor households, the economic burden of TB leads to reduced consumption, sale of assets, and greater debt, all of which result in further impoverishment, and often, destitution.

How can the economic burden due to TB on the poor be reduced?

Based on the available evidence and global experiences, India's Tuberculosis Control Programme can create more programmes to support TB patients in need. India has launched numerous direct transfers of money programmes, but many of these remain inaccessible due to lack of information, ineffective execution, and systemic problems. These consist of cash paid as part of a social security system or a programme incentive, transport reimbursements, treatment allowances and the like that are paid directly to affected individuals to ensure they do not become desperately poor or fall into debt. In most cases, these payments remain nominal. All individuals with active TB should receive a periodic assessment of their nutritional status and appropriate counselling based on their nutritional status, starting at diagnosis and continuing throughout their treatment. If unable to afford appropriate nutrition, they should be provided with locally available nutrient-rich or fortified supplementary foods to restore normal nutritional status. Food assistance improves access and adherence to treatment and mitigates the financial and social consequences of TB. While some of these plans are in existence in some Indian states these need to be expanded nationwide and the payments handed out under them need to be increased.

What is the role of community-based care system, skill development, and financial assistance in fighting TB?

Clinic-based treatment supervision places a significant economic burden on patients. Also, poor geographical and financial access to health services often prevent or delay medical help-seeking among people with TB. The creation or strengthening of community-based treatment supervision programmes would have the greatest potential impact on reducing patients' TB-related costs. Also, expansion of adherence technologies such as 99 DOTS can create more empowered systems of care where patients are allowed independence to manage their treatment. Training programmes or credits that help individuals or families affected by TB to generate income after treatment are crucial. This is particularly relevant for TB-affected people who work in the informal sector and lose employment due to the disease. This ensures that families and individuals are able to rebuild their lives and do not fall into poverty due to TB.

(Sourced from Survivors Against TB, SATB)

www.ingramcontent.com/pod-product-compliance
Lightning Source LLC
LaVergne TN
LVHW041929070526
838199LV00051BA/2764